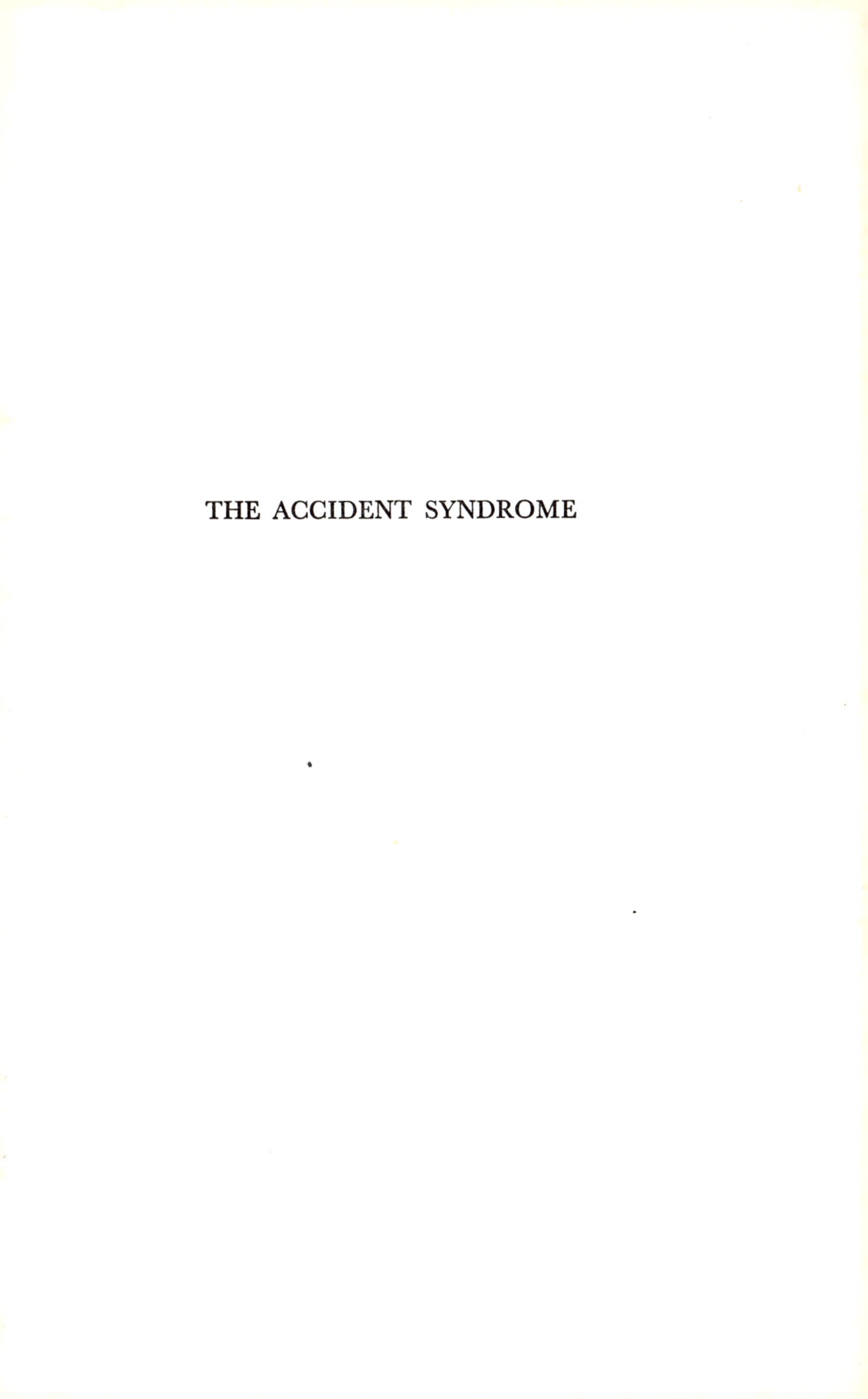

THE ACCIDENT SYNDROME

THE ACCIDENT SYNDROME

The Genesis of Accidental Injury

A CLINICAL APPROACH

By

MORRIS S. SCHULZINGER, M.A., M.D.

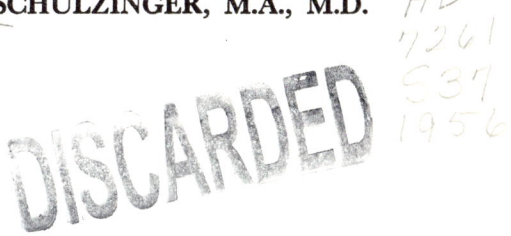

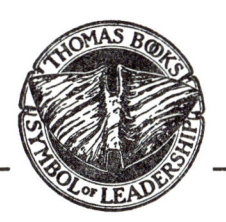

CHARLES C THOMAS · PUBLISHER
Springfield · Illinois · U.S.A.

CHARLES C THOMAS • PUBLISHER
BANNERSTONE HOUSE
301-327 East Lawrence Avenue, Springfield, Illinois, U.S.A.

Published simultaneously in the British Commonwealth of Nations by
BLACKWELL SCIENTIFIC PUBLICATIONS, LTD., OXFORD, ENGLAND

Published simultaneously in Canada by
THE RYERSON PRESS, TORONTO

This book is protected by copyright. No part of it may be reproduced in any manner without written permission from the publisher.

Copyright, 1956, by CHARLES C THOMAS • PUBLISHER

Library of Congress Catalog Card Number: 55-11250

Printed in the United States of America

To

Rachel, Peninah, Judith and Joseph

PREFACE

Few physicians and possibly no hospitals, have available detailed accidental injury records in large numbers compiled by one individual over a score of years. Somewhat on an unplanned basis over the period of 1930-1948, one physician painstakingly compiled the details of the social and medical background connected with some thirty-five thousand consecutive accidental injuries. By no means do these thirty-five thousand injuries represent thirty-five thousand individuals, since an essence of the worth of this material relates to the multiplicity of accidents in the total population that provided these informations. On a fortunate basis these records were compiled on a somewhat stable population within which this physician medically served large numbers of industrial workers in nearby small plants, but at the same time was their family physician. A single set of appraising standards was directed to the lifelong background of individuals who suffered injury at work, in the home, on the highways and at play.

These medical records were not compiled for any predetermined, unified purpose and certainly not for the project to which admirably they lent themselves a score of years after their inception. Day by day they were assembled solely for the purposes of good individual medical historics, many in the handwriting of the one physician whose conceptions pervaded the entire lot.

Twenty years after the beginning of these one-man records, it became apparent that therein existed a gross series of unique medical data from which might be extracted large or small samples for statistical examination.

This first delving into these thirty-five thousand consecutive accidental injury records is concerned with the ultimate causation of accidental injury. The proximate accident episode was deemed to be, in the greater number of accidents, only the culmination of a train of events long presaging an accident with or without injury or a series of such happenings. These records under investigation in great fidelity supplied the historical background, often well revealing the ultimate causation of the injury that brought together physician and patient.

During the half century period just now completed, the notable achievements in the prevention of accidents centered about mechanical devices both in and out of industry and in procedures and practices related to machinery and other operations providing some threat to operators and others in the vicinity. The reduction in accidents from the reliance upon mechanical devices and training is outstanding and soundly is proved. By this time it has become apparent that the limit of protective services from such efforts alone is in sight and that as to the future, no striking betterment as to accident frequency or severity may be expected. The law of diminishing returns has operated to this end and yet accidents in industry, in the home and on the highway continue with distressing frequency. By admission of those working in the field of safety, a continuation of these efforts at best only could eliminate about ten per cent of the now remaining accident episodes.

The second phase of major effort toward accident reduction was directed toward the education of those exposed, whether in the factory, home or in travel. It is not possible or needful to designate the time in which this approach was inaugurated. Manifestly from the beginning of the human race warnings toward safety precautions might have been heard. Nor would it be helpful, even though possible, to fix any period in which this type of effort culminated, if indeed by the present time it has culminated. The objective of this comment is to register the obvious that the enormous effort expended in safety education has not yielded results proportional to that effort. It now is clear that new approaches are in order if further major reduction in accident occurrence is to be achieved. The fecund opportunity appears to reside in the mind, behavior, habits, physical status, environment and inheritance of all persons to whom accidents may befall, which category of course embraces all persons.

Certainly it is no new concept that the accident victim more often than not is a direct contributor in the accident occurrence. What is new, or at least newer, is the realization that this background, out of

PREFACE

which accidents arise, strikingly is individualistic. Little can be detected by any mass approach and scarcely anything is to be eradicated by educative measures directed to groups. More and more it becomes apparent, and troublesomely so, that added achievements in accident prevention more than ever before must deal with the individual, his family, his environment and his behavior. The new opportunity in accident prevention strikingly becomes medical and the need is for an integrated clinical approach. This approach lends itself to some eighty per cent or ninety per cent of these accidents that now remain, after the mighty reductions related to mechanical safety procedures and the nearly equal victories resulting from mass education.

Without debate from any quarter, it will be recognized that of all accidents, some ten to twenty per cent are brought about solely on the basis of fortuity and in which the victim made no contribution whatever as to causation. The injured passenger in a railroad wreck was not conceivably a contributor to the causation of the catastrophe. Equally so the individual who is struck by a dislodged flowerpot while walking properly on the sidewalk in front of a tall building is nowise to be labeled as a sharer in the production of his injury. Instead, in the conceptions of this book, the individuals possibly in need of the medical approach were in the first instance the railroad engineer or his train dispatcher, and in the second, the reckless apartment resident who foolishly stored flowerpots on the window ledge. This book has no direct concern in these ten per cent to twenty per cent of all accidental injuries solely occurring under circumstances of fortuity. This book is concerned with appraisal of the remaining eighty per cent to ninety per cent of accidental injuries or accidents without injury in which unerringly may be traced the role of the victim in provoking his own misfortune.

The pattern that emerges from the totality of the statistical background becomes such a unity that the term, "the accident syndrome," becomes a verity. This syndrome of recurring manifestation and features takes on a quality of rigidity or at least substantiality. Only the details vary, but these variables become almost as numerous as the total number of individuals involved. This book undertakes the portrayal of the accident syndrome.

The years of exploration of this mass of statistical material of which this present book is only a small portion has led to debts of gratitude to the many who have joined in the exploration.

In this work an attempt is made to integrate into a meaningful whole the efforts and insights of such diverse disciplines as psychiatry, psychology, clinical medicine, social science, personnel management, safety engineering, industrial hygiene, education and safety. Personality, emotional, environmental and temporal factors all receive due weight and emphasis resulting in a tridimensional treatment of a most difficult subject. The volume is abundantly documented from the author's own studies and from other sources and supplies a basic tool for anyone who has professional or intellectual concern with the phenomenon of accidents. The clinical approach herein expounded gives rise to the constructive hypothesis that accident control lies in an understanding of the life factors of the whole person, rather than in an atomistic approach to the special hazards of his work and play environments. This volume literally fills a void and is intended for the professional groups concerned as well as for the interested lay reader. It is hoped that it will help disspel some of the obscurity, mysticism and taboos in which accidents are still largely enshrouded. But if it should do not more than inspire the intensive study of accidents at their point of origin, the individual human being, it shall be eminently worth-while.

M.S.S.

INTRODUCTION

THE study of accidents leading to an organized body of knowledge largely is the product of the present century. However, awareness of the peculiar significance of accidental injury is as old as man's recorded history. Did not the ancient Mosaic Law provide this injunction as to accident prevention? "When thou buildest a new house, then thou shalt make a battlement for thy roof, that thou bring not blood upon thy house, if any man fall from thence."

THE NUMBER OF ACCIDENTAL INJURIES

Scarcely is it within the accepted responsibility of this publication to emphasize the actuality of injury occurrence—the numbers of fatalities, permanent disability, temporary disability, etc. No less, a single group of figures here supplied should afford conviction of what is known to all—the enormous numbers of accidental injuries.

TABLE 1.4

PRINCIPAL CLASSES OF ACCIDENTS IN 1951

(71) (*National Safety Council*)

Classes	Total Deaths	Rate	Disabling Injuries
1. Motor Vehicle	37,300	24.3	1,350,000
2. Home	28,000	18.3	4,250,000
3. Occupation	16,000	10.4	2,100,000
4. Public (non-motor vehicle)	15,000	9.8	1,900,000
Total	96,300		9,600,000

In 1951, off-the-job injuries resulted in a loss of sixty million man-days of work; while on-the-job injuries resulted in a loss of fifty million man-days directly and 230 million man-days indirectly.

No figures of the type here presented are likely to embrace the highly numerous trivial injuries below the level leading to any medical care or for that matter any particular notice on the part of the victim. Commonly it is believed that for every injury at the level calling for medical care, some ninety-nine others arise falling into the category of the "trifling."

ACCIDENT WITHOUT HUMAN INJURY

The terms "accident" and "injury" have become so intertwined that the two are synonymous. But by no means does an accident necessarily lead to a personal injury. All of the requirements of an acceptable definition for an accident are fulfilled in the absence of any necessity for personal injury. It becomes clear that the driver whose automobile leaves the road, demolishes a barrier and perhaps rolls over one or more times, is involved in an accident. The fact that he was not injured does not in any wise destroy the fact of an accident's occurrence. On a psychological basis, as will be presented at later points, an accident without injury may provide all of the psychological requirements and satisfaction that provoked the accident in the first place. To a degree, personal injury associated with an accident is but a complication, but this complication assumes the position of the outstanding sequence in the happening. Moreover, personal injury may be requisite to the psychological situation over and over to be mentioned in this text. Throughout these discussions "accident" and "injury" are not the same, but the language encountered nearly always will disclose whether accident without injury or instead accidental personal injury is under contemplation.

WHAT IS AN ACCIDENT? WHAT IS AN ACCIDENTAL INJURY?

The term "accident" variously has been defined and carries many connotations and implications. In the field of practical safety and prevention, an accident presently and simply is defined as a suddenly occurring, unplanned, unintentional event which leads to personal injury or property damage.

This definition, as does many another, leans heavily upon the concept of "suddenly occurring." At once the absence of simplicity begins to appear. At least in legal appraisals an accident may be brought about under some conditions of prolonged exposure. Thus an accident may be caused when a person breathes over a period of hours a low concentration of carbon monoxide gas, which gas in time leads to a sufficient saturation of the blood to induce unconsciousness. At that moment it will become apparent to any observer that an accident usually unplanned, has taken place. Yet the time involved, which may have been as much as six to eight hours, undeniably properly may not be associated with the word "sudden." Like examples are abundant. In truth in some compensation insurance circles, it is the practice to regard any exposure leading to personal damage that operates for any less time than a full work period as constituting an accidental injury. If, however, the exposure period extends beyond one day's work hours, the ensuing body response may, at least at times, be termed an occupational disease.

In tracing the evolution of the term accident, the Encyclopedia Britannica (67) furnishes this statement:

"The kinship between what is 'essential' and what is necessary has prompted the common use of 'accident' for what is otherwise called 'chance' occurrence; and by a somewhat similar extension of its meaning the term 'accident' has come to be applied in law to any occurrence or result that could not have been foreseen by the agent, or to a result not designed (and therefore presumably not foreseen), and lastly, to anything unexpected."

The psychologist, Arbous, (7) "defines" an accident as follows:

"In a chain of events, each of which is planned or controlled, there occurs an unplanned event, which, being the result of some non-adjustive act on the part of the individual (variously caused) may or may not result in injury. This is an accident."

The author's definition of an accident is:

"An accident, with or without injury, is in the main a morbid phenomenon resulting from the integration of a dynamic variable constellation of forces and occurs as a sudden, unplanned and uncontrolled event."

It is to this definition, at least in its substance that adherence throughout this text is espoused.

ACCIDENT PRONENESS

Regardless of the acceptability of any definition of an "accident," currently much attention is directed to the notion that in any work group only a small number is to be identified with a high percentage of the total number of accidents that arise in any given period of time such as a month or year. It is easy to encounter the published statement that twenty per cent of any group of individuals, such as a factory population, may be found to be involved in some fifty-five per cent to eighty-five per cent of all accidents. This alleged accident proneness frequently is labeled as inherent and those so labeled acquire a stigmatization. This serious matter of accident proneness will be suitably pursued in the development of this text. Its mention at this point becomes inevitable, since the implications of accident proneness enter into and modify some definitions of "accidents." Some analytical psychiatrists view most accidents as subconsciously purposeful acts along with pain, damage or loss, bringing to the victim a variety of psychological gains and thus serving the psychic economy. It will now become apparent that at least on the subconscious level some accidents are not "unplanned," not "unintentional," and thus is upset the simplicity of even the best definition of an accident. It is the thesis of this text that inherent accident proneness scarcely exists, while fleeting or mildly prolonged accident proneness is widespread.

THE RESPONSIBILITY FOR ACCIDENTS

At this moment the term "responsibility" stands in no relationship to legal responsibility, monies for property damage, fines, etc. Instead, the responsibility appraised relates to the attitude of the producer of the accident, having in mind the utter unwillingness of many an accident producer to identify himself in any degree with the accident causation. The concept of an "accident" as an untoward event resulting in damage to property or person to which the individual bears no responsibility largely is a product of our modern civilization. Primitive man accepted full responsibility for his mishaps and offered no alibis. In a measure this may mark him as our superior. However, primitive man was quite willing to associate his misfortune as punishment for his misdeeds or sinful behavior, as an act of God, as bad "luck," as warnings of major disasters or merely as carelessness. No less, primitive man identified himself with all of these explanations, since in that early time no psychologist intervened in absolving him from responsibility.

HUMAN FAILURE IN ACCIDENT AND ACCIDENT INJURY

Earlier it has been asserted that a plateau has been reached with respect to accident reduction growing out of the initial and admirable enterprises centering about such items as guards, goggles and gloves. Less in evidence is the plateau now visible as to accident frequency and severity reduction achieved through slogans, campaigns and educative devices. Certainly no disdain attends the measures mentioned. In fact, so successful have they been in industry that the frequency locus of injury no longer is in the factory but the home, the highway and the sports area. Wherever accidents arise, it becomes apparent that the promising fruitful preventive attack is concerned with human failings such as haste, inattention, preoccupation, distraction, which in turn may relate to emotional strain or conflict resulting from anxiety, anger, fear, frustration, hate, aggression and guilt. Thus a newly detected factor in the etiology of accidents has been added, the personality factor—the contribution arising from within the individual—an intrinsic contribution born of emotional strain or conflict temporary or inherent within the individual. Since stigma is likely to be incurred by any investigator who emphasizes "newness," it may be well fully to grant the lack of complete "newness" in emphasizing the abnormal personality factor in accident causation. What newness there is chiefly resides in the recognition that a new direction has been provided. This new direction, however definite in its prospects of affording an opportunity for major reduction in accidents, unfortunately is not one that may be invaded as freely or as successfully as characterized the early decades of safety protection. For the first time accident prevention demands the professional attainments of medical personnel. Less attention will be directed to the concept of the "human machine" and more directed to the significance of behavior deviation brought about in the realm of the frailties of the mind.

THE ACCIDENT SYNDROME

The analysis of the thirty-five thousand consecutive accidental injury records that constitute the material in hand for appraisal, along with the rich literature devoted to the genesis of accidental injury, yields the tangibility that this new direction in accident causation exploration is associated with an accident syndrome. This syndrome is not entirely the usual medical recurrence of signs and symptoms, although medical signs and symptoms are involved. Instead, it is a syndrome in the larger sense of any frequently recurring items in a series. In this larger sense, the genesis of accidents is revealed as a series of detectable recurrences that pave the way for the prediction of accident probability wherever the essential elements of the syndrome are encountered.

In the foregoing the content, objectives and approaches of this text are presaged.

ACKNOWLEDGMENTS

INDEBTEDNESS is acknowledged to Dr. I. Arthur Mirsky, formerly Director of the May Research Institute of the Cincinnati Jewish Hospital, and Associate Professor of Experimental Medicine and Psychiatry at the University of Cincinnati, and now Professor and Chairman of the Department of Clinical Science and Professor of Experimental Psychiatry at the University of Pittsburgh, who first suggested the study of accident causation and for his encouragement and enthusiastic review of the original manuscript.

Dr. Donald Ross, Associate Professor of Psychiatry at University of Cincinnati, spent many hours in discussing the original research material and findings and was helpful in many other ways; Dr. D. J. Lauer, formerly Assistant Professor of Industrial Medicine at the University of Cincinnati and the Cincinnati Post-Graduate School of Industrial Medicine and the Kettering Laboratories and now Medical Director of Jones and Laughlin Steel Corporation commented appreciatively on the merits of the early manuscript; Dr. Herbert B. Weaver, formerly Professor of Psychology, University of Cincinnati and now Professor of Psychology and Head of the Department at the University of Hawaii was most helpful in the statistical analysis of the research data; Dr. Maurice Levine, Professor and Head of the Department of Psychiatry, University of Cincinnati, gave valuable grounding and orientation in psychiatric concepts; and Dr. Milton Rosenbaum, formerly Associate Professor of Psychiatry, University of Cincinnati and now Professor and Head of the Department of Psychiatry at the Albert Einstein College of Medicine, New York, made some valuable suggestions.

Especially, gratitude is expressed to Dr. Robert A. Kehoe, Professor of Industrial Medicine and Director of the Kettering Laboratory and the Post-Graduate School of Industrial Medicine, University of Cincinnati, for review and suggestions on the early manuscripts; to Dr. Frank Princi, Professor of Industrial Medicine,

University of Cincinnati, and editor of the *A.M.A. Archives of Industrial Health,* for his critical review of several interim manuscripts, for his encouragement and for many constructive suggestions; to Dr. Phillip Drinker, Professor Department of Industrial Hygiene, Harvard School of Public Health and chief editor of the *A.M.A. Archives of Industrial Health* for review of several interim manuscripts; to Dr. Fay M. Hemphill, Associate Professor of Public Health, School of Public Health, University of Michigan, for aid in the selection, review and analysis of the statistical material; to Dr. Carey P. McCord, Consultant, Institute of Industrial Health, University of Michigan and editor of *Industrial Medicine and Surgery* for editing the current manuscript and for many valuable suggestions, and to Mr. A. D. Cloud, publisher of *Industrial Medicine and Surgery,* who in sustained friendship and encouragement has paved the way for this book.

A debt of appreciation is owed to my present and former office assistants Mmes. Hilda Kroger Mattes, Katherine B. Lange, Izola Laster, Doris Schwendeman and Dr. and Mrs. Norman Straw for their generous help in assembling and typing some of the data and material; to Messrs. Nahum Marmet and Hirsch Horwitz and to my niece Miss Chana Slavita for help in preparation of charts and tables and proofreading; to Mr. Sam Feldman for statistical help; to Messrs. Max Singer, Lucien Cohen, J. Siegel and Drs. J. Stubbins and Joseph D. Weintraub for various courtesies.

I also owe a debt of gratitude to the editorial staff of the Charles C Thomas, Publisher, especially to Mr. Warren H. Green, for their patience and for the many kindnesses which I have received in the course of publication of this book; to Joseph B. Homan, Professor of Medical Art, College of Medicine, University of Cincinnati, and to Mmes. Margaret M. Cook and Hilde Beatty, for help with charts and drawings.

The company that joined in this statistical adventure and study, small though it be, is larger than these names just mentioned. For all the unnamed ones the appreciation is just as great. I alone am responsible for the facts and views presented in this book.

M.S.S.

CONTENTS

PREFACE	vii
INTRODUCTION	xi
The Number of Accidental Injuries	xi
Accident Without Human Injury	xii
What is an Accident? What Is an Accidental Injury?	xii
Accident Proneness	xiv
The Responsibility for Accidents	xiv
Human Failure in Accident and Accidental Injury	xv
The Accident Syndrome	xvi
ACKNOWLEDGEMENTS	xvii
THE ACCIDENT SYNDROME—FRONTISPIECE	2

Chapter

1.	WORK MATERIAL AND THE METHODS OF THEIR EXPLORATION	3
2.	MAJOR FINDINGS AND CONCLUSIONS	11
	General	11
	Time, Season, Weather	11
	Age	12
	Sex	12
	Proneness, Repetition	13
	Maladjustment	14
	Cause	15
	Fortuity	16
	Frequency	16
	Daily Number of Accidents	16
	Body Area	16
	Epidemics of Accidents	17
	The Accident Syndrome	17
	Comment on Conclusions	18
	Age	18
	Sex	19
	Age and sex distribution in illness compared to accidents	20

Multiple or repeated accidents 21
The incidence of accidents in irresponsible and
    maladjusted individuals 23
The incidence of accidents in relation to the annual cycle 26
Incidence by months 26
Seasonal incidence of accidents 28
The incidence of accidents in relation to the
    diurnal cycle 29
Hourly distribution of repeated accidents 33

3. CONCEPTS OF ACCIDENT CAUSATION 34
   1. Introduction and History 34
   2. Psychodynamics 41
   3. Psychodynamics of Accidents in Children 55

4. CHARTS AND TABLES 60
   Charts
     Cases from Handling Household Utensils by Age and Sex 61
     Cases from Handling Objects by Age and Sex 62
     Cases from Falls by Age and Sex 63
     Cases from Aggression by Age and Sex 64
     Cases from Aggression by Age, in Groups A and B 65
     Cases from Foreign Bodies by Age and Sex 66
     Cases from Motor Vehicles by Age and Sex 67
     Cases from Stumbling by Age and Sex 68
     Month and Season of Accidents by Age and Sex 69
     Hours of Accidents by Age and Sex 79
     Accidents by Age and Sex in Relation to
        Cincinnati's Population 87
     Industrial Accidents by Age in Relation to
        Cincinnati's Employed Population 89
     Non-Industrial Accidents by Age and Sex 90
     Multiple Accidents by Age in Groups A and B 91
     Number of Persons Injured and Number of
        Accidents per Person 93
     Illness from All Causes by Age and Sex 94
     Accidents by Age and Sex 95
     Multiple Accidents by Age and Sex in Groups A and B 96
     Cases from Motor Vehicles by Age and Sex in
        Groups A and B 100

Single and Multiple Accidents, by Sex, in
Groups A and B ... 103

Tables

Industrial Accidents by Age and Sex ... 106
Accidents by Age, Sex, and Groups A and B ... 107
Principal Classes of Accidents in 1951 ... 109
Principal Types or Means of Accidents in 1951 ... 109
Principal Classes of Accidents Among Workers in 1951 ... 109
Types of Injury by Age and Sex, in Groups A and B ... 110
Parts of Body Injured, by Age and Sex,
in Groups A and B ... 113
Types of Accidents by Age, in Groups A and B ... 117
Principal Means of Accidents, Extent of Severity
and Disability ... 119
Causes of Hospitalized Home Accidents ... 120
Industrial and Non-Industrial Accidents by Month ... 120
Non-Industrial Accidents by Month ... 121
Seasonal Distribution of Industrial Accidents ... 122
Single Industrial Accidents by Month and Age ... 122
Multiple Industrial Accidents by Month and Age ... 122
Single and Multiple Industrial Accidents by Month and Age ... 123
Incidence of Accidents by Month ... 123
Half and Quarter Day Frequency of Industrial and
Non-Industrial Accidents by Sex ... 124
Hour of Non-Industrial Accidents by Age and Sex ... 125
Hourly Per Cent Distribution of Total Accident Cases ... 125
Hour of Industrial Accidents ... 126
Six-Hourly Groupings of Single and Multiple
Non-Industrial Accidents by Sex and Groups A and B ... 132
Hour of Day and Season of Year of
Non-Industrial Accidents ... 133
Industrial Accidents by Sex in Two-Hour Periods ... 134
Percentage of Industrial and Non-Industrial Accident
Patients by Place of Residence ... 135
Industrial Accidents by Types of Industry and Sex ... 135
Industrial Accidents by Number of Accidents
Per Firm and Number of Firms ... 136
Percentage of Non-Industrial and Industrial Injuries
in Relation to Cincinnati's Population ... 136

Single and Multiple Industrial Accidents by Sex in
  Single Year Groups..137
Industrial Patients with Single and Multiple Accidents
  by Sex 138
Non-Industrial Patients with Multiple Accidents in
  Groups A and B...139
Cumulative Percentage of Industrial Single and
  Multiple by Sex and Age...140
Single and Multiple Industrial Accidents by Age,
  Year and Sex...141
Industrial Patients by Sex, Age and Number of Accidents......142
Percentage of Single and Multiple Industrial
  Accidents by Age and Year..143
Ratio of Number of Accidents to Number of Patients
  by Year and Sex..144
Non-Industrial Patients by Number of Injuries, Sex and Age..145
Industrial Patients by Number of Injuries, Sex and Age..........146
Industrial Patients Having Single or Multiple Accidents
  in Two or More Consecutive Years......................................146
Industrial Patients Having Single or Multiple Accidents
  in Any Two or More Years in a Six-Year Period................146
Frequency of Recurrence of Multiple Accidents in the
  Same Industrial Patients in Three-Year Periods.................147
Multiple Non-Industrial Accidents by Age and Sex
  and Groups A and B...148
Non-Industrial Patients by Age, Sex and Number of
  Accidents in Groups A and B...149
Frequency Distribution of Six Hundred Forty-Seven
  Industrial Accidents According to Number of Ac-
  cidents Per Patient Compared with Three Theo-
  retical Possibilities 150
Observed and Theoretical Distribution of Accidents................150
Mean Accident Frequency of a Group of Shunters
  During Three One-Year Periods of Obesrvation,
  and the Effect of Removing Workers with the
  Highest Accident Frequency Rates on the Remain-
  der of the Group...151
Correlation Between Accidents in Two Consecutive
  Periods 151

CONTENTS

  Illness from All Causes, by Age and Sex, and
    Groups A and B 152
  Comparison of Percentage of Patients Having Multiple
    Accidents Between Group A and Group B 152
  Comparison of Age Distribution of Non-Industrial
    Accident Population with Cincinnati Census 153
  Correlation Between Hour of Occurrence of Industrial
    and Non-Industrial Injuries 154
  Correlation Between Age of Distributions of
    Selected Samples 155
  Differences Between Age Distribution of Various
    Accident Samples 156

5. THE ACCIDENT SYNDROME 160
  Universal Risk 161
  Irregular Additional Risk Incident to Physical Impairment 161
  Abnormal Physical Environment 162
  Maladjustment and Irresponsibility 164
  The Trigger Episode 168
  Behavior in the Presence of the Trigger Mechanism 169
  The Prospective Accident With or Without Injury 170

6. ACCIDENT PRONENESS 175

7. PSYCHOLOGICAL FACTORS IN ACCIDENT CAUSATION
  AND PREVENTION 180
  Accident Causation—In Review 182
  Accident Prevention 184

8. THE INCIDENCE OF ACCIDENTS IN IRRESPONSIBLE AND
  MALADJUSTED INDIVIDUALS 190

9. HEALTH AND HANDICAPS 195
  Physical Handicaps 200
  Mood Swings 202

10. THE CLINICAL MEDICAL APPROACH 206

11. SUMMATION 210

BIBLIOGRAPHY 219
INDEX 225

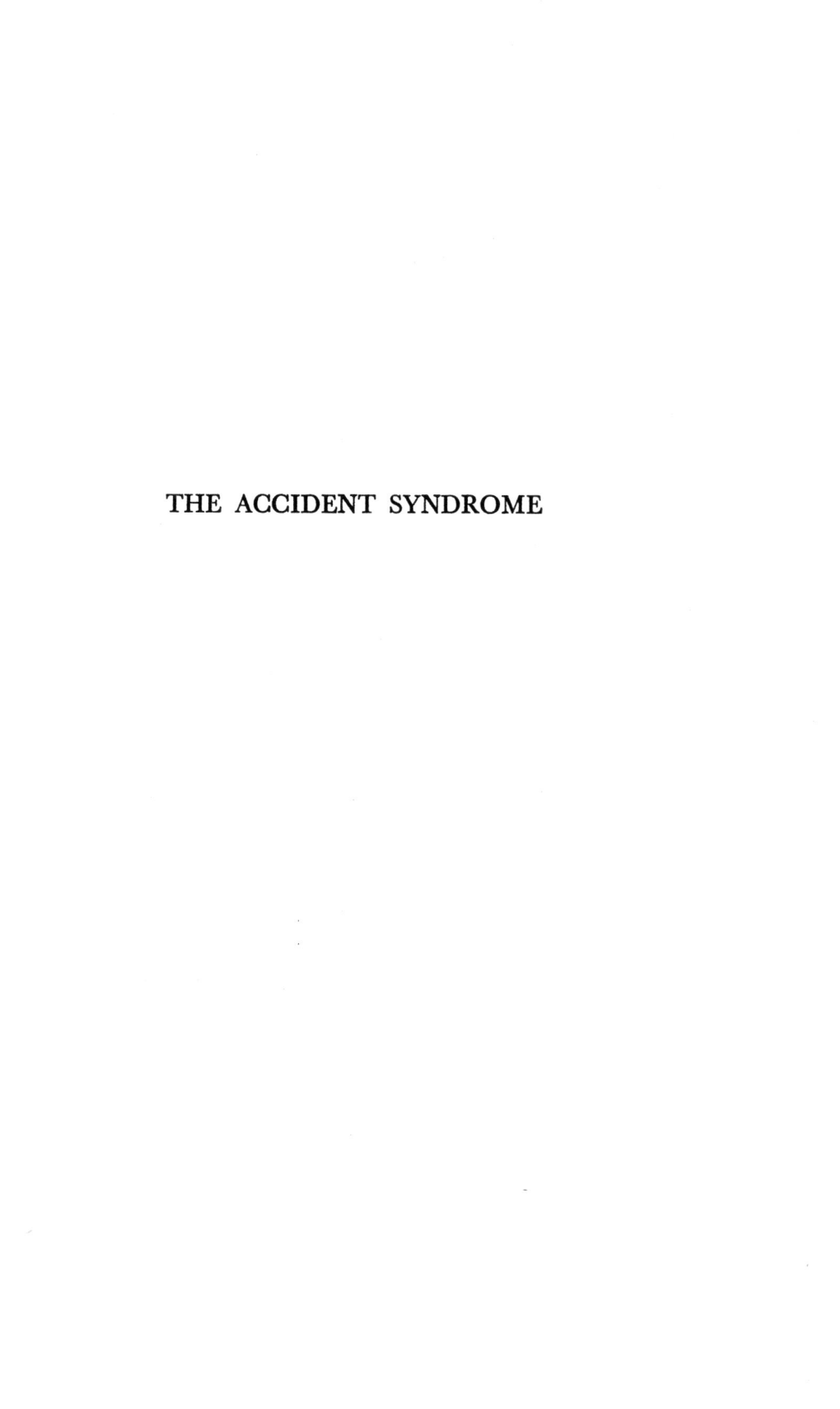

THE ACCIDENT SYNDROME

```
[Universal Risk] + [Abnormal physical environment] + [Maladjustment and Irresponsibility] + [The Trigger Episode] + [Behavior in the presence of the trigger]  →  [Accident with or without personal injury]
```

[Irregular additional risk incident to physical impairment] connects to [Abnormal physical environment]

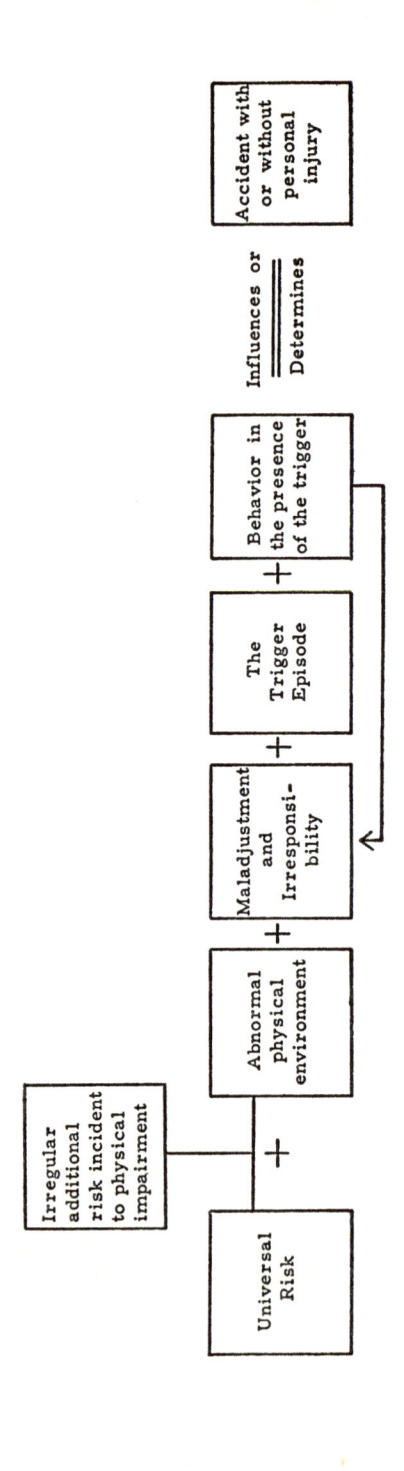

Influences or / Determines

THE ACCIDENT SYNDROME

Eighty to ninety per cent of all accidents present discernible contributory human causative factors.

CHAPTER ONE

WORK MATERIAL AND THE METHODS OF THEIR EXPLORATION

THE present contribution of new material to the total effort to clarify accident causation consists of various analyses of thirty-five thousand consecutive accident records in one physician's medical practice. This chapter describes this work material, the extent of analysis together with descriptions of the methods used in the exploration of these data.

From 1930 to 1948 some thirty-five thousand cases (thirty-four thousand eight hundred and seventy-two to be exact) of accidental injury were treated in a general medical practice in Cincinnati, Ohio. These thirty-five thousand instances of accidental injury involved twenty-seven thousand eight hundred and sixty-five individuals. However, this last figure is not exact, since through necessity some persons appear in two categories. Thus as will appear presently, one broad classification is confined to industrial injuries, another is concerned with non-industrial injuries. On occasion industrial workers may appear in those records devoted to industrial injuries, but otherwise be included in the non-industrial injuries when accidents occurred apart from gainful employment. This fact accounts for occasional apparent discrepancies in records when in fact no real discrepancy exists. Obviously the total number of individuals involved will never attain to the total number of injuries, since many patients over the years were treated for numerous injuries.

This work material was divided into three categories now to be described. Group A provided five thousand two hundred and forty-one accident injury records involving four thousand eight hundred and forty-six individuals. This group includes individuals of all ages from infancy to senility. The industrial injury group provided the records of twenty-seven thousand two hundred and thirty-five cases and twenty thousand nine hundred and thirty-four individuals. Since all of the persons involved were adults, it follows that the age distribution in the industrial group would be distinctly different than in Group. A.

The population of Group B (two thousand three hundred and ninety-six accidents and two thousand eighty-five individuals) represents a selected sample deemed to include some but not all patients with some form of maladjustment. This group is described in some detail in Chapter Eight.

For the purposes of investigating accident frequency in relation to the incidence of sickness, three thousand illness instances were included. The majority of the individuals involved in the analyses in the records of illness are otherwise included in some one of the categories just described.

The usual medical history of minor injury records includes the recording of only limited information. Seldom do these records in hospitals and offices of private physicians include elaboration beyond the obviously required data including: age and sex of patient, circumstances of the immediate injury and its treatment. The records used in this series provide information on the following:

1. Place of residence
2. Sex, age.
3. Date and time of accidental occurrence.
4. Type of accident and extensive description of the accidental occurrence.
5. History of previous accidents.
6. Location of person at time of accident.
7. Status of person's activity at the time of accident, whether gainfully employed.
8. Usual occupation.

The medical examination records included:

1. Body site of injury.
2. Nature and extent of injury.

Data from these sources were organized under many and various categories, for example:

1. Industrial (during course of gainful employment) and non-industrial.
2. Place of accident such as: home, farm, school, public, industrial, plant. etc.

3. Time of occurrence by year, month, day of week and hour of day.
4. Usual residence of patient.
5. Frequency of injuries to the same person (multiple accidents).

Studies were carried out on such single characteristics as these and, in addition, the data often were arranged into designs for evaluation of relative effects of the various factors. Examples of statistical methods of such evaluation are included in the Chapter Charts and Tables.

The cases of the series are perhaps representative of those in many general practitioners' experiences. Many plants and business establishments of Cincinnati are included, but the cases are not limited to industrial accidents. Those which were classified industrial include diversified occupations, age groups, types of injuries and like categories. Various social, economic and cultural levels are included in the series. Some fifty per cent of the non-industrial patients and thirteen per cent of the industrial group resided in the neighborhood of the office, while the others lived in various sections of greater Cincinnati and surrounding rural communities. The series contains records on many family groups over many consecutive years, as well as patients seen only once or a few times and over limited time periods. Cases involving state compensation or public liability are present in the series along with the private pay and indigent patients. Such heterogenicity of patients is common among general physicians.

Comparative studies between the series and the Federal Census involving sex and age characteristics were made with the expected conclusion that the series is not representative of Cincinnati's population with regard to sex and age.

This description of the source and scope of the series provides an insight into their potential usefulness. Most studies of accidents which have been reported in the literature are based on experiences in major industry and, to a lesser extent, on traffic and other selective classes of accidents. There are relatively few studies of accidents in small industry. Yet sixty per cent of all industrial workers are employed in small plants and are involved in the majority of all industrial accidents. About eighty per cent of all the accidents in the United States now occur outside of industrial establishments. Therefore, the present study should be of special appeal because it is based on large samples of accidents in small industry and outside of industry.

Although this study has unique characteristics, it does not constitute a complete epidemiology of accidents. An ideal approach to the epidemiology of accidents should be based on the current accident histories of statistically significant groups of persons from birth until death. The series should represent a cross section of the entire population in relation to age and sex, their social, economic, cultural, vocational and marital status, as well as their ethnic origin and religious persuasion. Furthermore, studies of accident frequency should record near misses, accidents which result only in damage to property, in injury to other persons, in trivial injuries, as well as those which result in fractures, disabling injuries and other serious or fatal injuries. The physical, mental and emotional state of the accident patient and a variety of factors in the external environment also are of significance. Such an ideal study obviously is unobtainable. Of necessity, we must limit ourselves to the study of accident series which are "biased" or selective in some respects and allow for the shortcomings.

The concern with near misses, with accidents that result in property damage only, and with trivial injuries, is based on the findings that, while the incidence of accidents is frequently related to personality or psychological factors, the presence or absence of injury following an accident, as well as the severity of the injury, are frequently determined by the presence or absence of, or the nature of, environmental hazards, or by chance factors.

Over long periods of time, the remembered histories of accidents are usually limited to fractures and other serious injuries. Because of the common difficulty in recalling accidents, a patient's memory is an unreliable index to the true incidence of injury. He frequently will deny previous accidents, when numerous scars on exposed areas are mute witnesses to his true accident history. The memory of accidents may be erased rapidly because of their trivial nature or because their recall may evoke feelings of guilt, anxiety or pain.

As a result of differences in cultural background, economic status and psychological needs, there is often little relationship between the incidence of injury and the number of accidents which receive medical attention. Individuals with identical life histories of accidents may have entirely different recorded or remembered histories. One may have many recorded as well as remembered histories, while the other may have few or none. The recorded as well as the remembered accident histories may thus register the patient's attitude toward his injuries or accidents and not the actual number of his accidents. In some respects, the given history of accidents is not unlike a given history of colds. The patient remembers that he has had colds, or those colds that are of special significance to him, but will seldom remember the number of colds.

All this is illustrated in a cited instance:

Mr. H. H., age thirty-seven, a steel construction foreman, presents himself for treatment of an injury to his left ankle which he sustained on a Sunday at home two weeks earlier, when he fell down a flight of stairs. He is six feet two inches tall, weighs two hundred and twenty pounds, is intelligent, serene, calm, unhurried, unworried, earns more than $100 a week, has a wife and two small children and appears to be a well balanced and well adjusted individual.

Examination reveals a swollen, discolored ankle and a spiral fracture of the distal end of the fibula. The patient has not lost any time from work during the two weeks that have elapsed since the injury, in spite of a considerable amount of pain. He sought medical advice only because the injury did not heal in what he considered to be a reasonable length of time. When questioned about his past history, the patient stated that he had never had an injury before, that he lives a happy life at home and at work and does not have a thing to worry about. In the course of casual conversation the following story is elicited:

"Of course, I have had many scratches and bruises. Oh, yes. I had a fractured jaw when I was seventeen; I was kicked by a mule on the chin. I also had a sprained ankle when I was twenty-one, soon after I got married."

"Any other injuries?"

"Oh, well, I fell down a couple of floors several times; only got some scratches and bruises, you know; that doesn't count."

"Was I ever hurt when I was a little boy? Come to think of it, a doctor did sew me up, the left side of my 'stomach,' when I was five."

The conversation then turned to the patient's life experiences and eagerly he related that he was the eldest of five siblings, that he was born and raised in a fairly prosperous Kentucky farm home in a coal-mining district. He started working in the mines when he was quite young, was trapped twice in mine catastrophies and remained alive each time only with some hours to spare. He witnessed many horrible, mutilating and fatal accidents. There were numerous accidents among uncles and other close relatives, but there were few to speak of in his own immediate family. In spite of the narrow escapes and horrifying experiences, the patient looked back with a feeling of nostalgia to his life as a miner. "It was exciting and thrilling," he said, "always something new and, of course, it requires a great deal of skill and ingenuity to be a miner."

It may be well to recall that the patient's first response was that previously he had never had an accident. The above history was elicited as a result of patient, time-consuming effort. Given more time, a more elaborate accident history undoubtedly would have been obtained.

This single item reflects the character of the approach that has attended the compilation of the records that have led to this book. The epidemiology of accidents has been studied from a variety of "samples" or "universes." Among these may be mentioned factory, home, automobile, or public accidents; hospital records, insurance mortality records and home surveys. Each of these "universes" has a selective quality or "bias" of its own. Accident statistics, no matter how carefully compiled, are seldom free from "bias."

The writer's series of accidents are selective, among other things, on the basis of the patient's decision to seek medical aid, the choice of physician, the lack of full information on the nature and number of all of the patient's previous accidents and the lack of a parent population suited for control purposes.

Many of the accident patients who came to the author's clinic for the treatment of their accidents had such trivial injuries, ones that they easily could have treated themselves or left untreated. This experience is shared by most physicians. The seeking of medical aid thus denotes the degree of significance which the patient attributes to the particular accident, the injury, and/or the "benefit" of being treated by a physician. The factor determining whether an accident patient applies for medical aid thus frequently is not the severity of the injury, but the patient's state of emotional equilibrium and his need for a relationship therapy by a physician, that is, his surrogate father or mother.

Despite the size of the present series, some of the sub-studies would be more convincing if the samples were larger and better controlled. In the final analysis, it is through the comparative studies of many samples by different observers that one is able to differentiate between the truly valid and the invalid and also between those facts which lend themselves to generalization and those which only hold true for the given culture, locality or sample.

Prior to presentation of the examples, some explanation is needed for statistical treatment of these data beyond the mere presentation of tables of frequency and percentages as usually employed in medical publications. Suppose an arrangement is made showing the frequency and percentage of the population of Cincinnati by age groups: (1) taken from data collected during a decennial census, and (2) likewise for the series of cases for the same year. Then, consider the problem as: "Does the sample represent the population of Cincinnati in its age characteristics?" or stated differently, "If a random sample of the population of Cincinnati were selected of the size of this series of cases, with what probability could it be expected that the sample would be distributed by age like the series with which we are dealing?" Certainly, by comparing the percentages visually, differences are obvious, but direct comparison of percentages provides an insufficient answer to the specific problem. However, there exist relatively simple mathematical devices that afford promise of rigid tests for the problem and which may be relatively easily applied in our specific situations. One such technique is known as the "Chi square test of goodness of fit." There are other statistical tests that might have been chosen to serve the same purpose, but this one was selected because of its simplicity and applicability. As a result of this brief test, we may conclude that the population in the accident series is distributed "significantly" differently by age from that of the population of Cincinnati (as measured.) We are assured that we risk being wrong in making this statement far less than one chance in a hundred. Truly, in this instance our risk is less than one in ten thousand, but we wish only to establish "levels" of risk and, arbitrarily, decided that probabilities of less than one in a hundred would be accepted as significant.

Another statistical application frequently used is that of the "critical ratio" which by some authors is called the "t" test. Its application is demonstrated in the chapter on Charts and Tables.

This procedure provides evidence of making a meaningful statement regarding the observed differences between two proportions (in this demonstration, between two percentages) and concluding, with assurance of being right in our conclusion more than ninety-nine in one hundred times, that the industrial group of our selected series is more prone to multiple accidents within a specified time period than is the non-industrial group.

A third common statistical tool employed is exemplified in a study to determine the extent and significance of correlation existing between frequency of occurrence of accidents as distributed by hour of occurrence for (1) the industrial group, and (2) the non-industrial group. This procedure of Rank Order Correlation is demonstrated in the Chapter on Charts and Tables.

These statistical procedures are simply quantitative and do not imply or designate any "reason" or "cause" for the existence of the quantitative relationships which they determine. Interpretations of causation must come from the experience and knowledge of those familiar with the field in which the data originate. Statistical techniques are a useful adjunct in clinical and other studies, but they are not a substitute for clinical experience and knowledge.

CHAPTER TWO

MAJOR FINDINGS AND CONCLUSIONS

The objectives of this book will not be served by the withholding to the point of the final chapter the oustanding observations, findings and conclusions that provide the core of this publication. Instead resort is had to that other device of early presentation of findings stated without elaboration in the hope that the mere presentation may provide a willingness to pursue their origin within the body of the publication. Operating on that basis it is observed:

GENERAL
Foremost in any tabulation of findings and conclusions is the observation that the circumstances attending causation of an accident with or without injury lend themselves to the construction or formulation of a syndrome with several components, chief of which is the mental maladjustment of the accident victim, temporary or prolonged, to his environment.

TIME, SEASON, WEATHER
Children under the age of fifteen have the most nearly perfect annual cyclical pattern of distribution of accidents, as well as the widest range of difference between the high incidence of summer and the low of winter; while the reverse is true at the opposite extreme of life.
The incidence of accidents follows a relatively fixed annual cyclical pattern of distribution; increasing steadily from a low in February to a high in June and August and then decreasing steadily to the low.
The incidence of accidents at its low in February is identical for both sexes and all age groups.
The incidence of non-industrial accidents follows a diurnal cyclical pattern of distribution, increasing from a low at 5:00 a.m. to a peak at 5:00 p.m.
The peak hour for accidents as well as the diurnal pattern of distribution of accidents vary with age and sex.
In children under the age of fifteen, the peak hour for accidents is 5:00

p.m.; between the ages of fifteen and forty it is 10-11 p.m.: in those forty years and older it is 3-5 p.m.

In industrial accidents, the peak hours for accidents are 10:00 a.m. and 3:00 p.m. (mid-morning and mid-afternoon) in day workers and the hours of 8:00 p.m. and 10:00 p.m. in night workers.

The causes of seasonal fluctuations of accident rates have not been fully determined. Climatic and seasonal stresses on body and spirit as well as a host of social and economic factors are probably important determinants.

The percentage of summer accidents decreases significantly with increment in age.

In children of school age (ages 6-15) the ratio of school-hour accidents (8:00 a.m. to 3:00 p.m.) to non-school-hour accidents remain unchanged during all seasons except in spring when there is a significant increase in the ratio of non-school-hour accidents.

AGE

Accidents are primarily an affliction of youth—fifty per cent occur before the age of twenty-five and seventy per cent before the age of thirty-five. The age of twenty-one is the peak year for accidents.

In children, the ages of two-four and eight are peak years for accidents. Girls have their lowest incidence of accidents at the age of thirteen and boys at the age of eleven.

The period of highest incidence of accidents begins at seventeen years of age and is virtually over at twenty-eight.

The range of difference between the high incidence of accidents in summer and the low incidence in winter narrows signficantly with increment in age.

SEX

Males have a significantly higher incidence of accidents than females during every year of the normal life span except the first.

Aggressive behavior accidents are predominantly more frequent in males, in irresponsible-maladjusted individuals and in the young of both sexes. Accidents are least likely to occur in a healthy young girl, age ten to fourteen, born and raised in a normally adjusted secure and loving home environment, during the winter months, the night hours and the home environment.

The diurnal distribution of accidents in female workers differs from that of male workers. In females, there is only one peak-hour for accidents,

10:00 a.m.; the morning accidents exceed the afternoon accidents; and there is a higher percentage of noon-hour accidents.

PRONENESS, REPETITION

Repeated accidents reach a peak of incidence at the age of five to nine years.

Most accidents are due to infrequent solitary experiences of large numbers of individuals.

Those treated for accidents during every year of three consecutive years account for a relatively small proportion (0.5%) of non-industrial accidents.

The tendency to have repeated accidents is a phenomenon that usually passes with age and is not a fixed trait of the individual.

Susceptibility to accidents and the experience of accidents are universal phenomena and most individuals are afflicted by accidents many times in the course of a lifetime.

The frequently reported observation that most accidents are due to a small fixed group of accident repeaters, commonly known as "accident-prone," holds true only when the period of observation is relatively short or when the numerical strength of the observed population greatly exceeds the numerical frequency of the accidents.

In the normally adjusted-responsible group, repeated accidents occur at a low and even rate through the age of fifty and then decrease steadily with increment in age.

Susceptibility to accidents, like susceptibility to illness, appears to be a problem in general morbidity. Individuals may be said to vary in their degree of susceptibility (or proneness) to accidents, rather than in the presence or absence of proneness.

Repeated accidents frequently occur during identical hours, especially in persons with a recorded history of three or more accidents.

Accidents often occur in chain fashion as if one accident acted as a trigger mechanism or as a sensitizing agent for another accident or series of accidents in the individual or the group.

In highly susceptible individuals, a series of repeated accidents may occur under the influence of increased stress or strain.

Most persons find solutions to their problems, develop defenses against their emotional conflicts and drop out of the highly "accident-prone" group after a few hours, days, weeks or months.

Some persons may remain highly susceptible to accidents throughout life, with or without lapses of years of freedom from the accident habit. These are the truly "accident-prone" individuals, they contribute, however, only a relatively small percentage of all the accidents.

The evidence indicates that, when the period of observation is sufficiently long, the "small group of persons who are responsible for most of the accidents" is essentially a shifting group of individuals with new persons constantly falling in and out of the group.

Despite a great deal of effort and the invention of a multitude of ingenious tests, "accident proneness" can be diagnosed, at present, only with the aid of a past history of multiple accidents.

A past history of repeated accidents is of itself not necessarily an indication of "accident proneness," hazardous exposure and other factors must be taken into account.

The accident habit is not necessarily a fixed quality. (Dunbar)

Accident-repeaters in one period tend to regress toward the average of the group in another period. (Cobb)

The ratio of male to female accidents is in the proportion of two to one; while repeated accidents are extremely rare in females.

Children of maladjusted-irresponsible families have a significantly higher incidence of accidents, especially multiple or repeated accidents, than children in normally adjusted-responsible families.

MALADJUSTMENT

Irresponsible and maladjusted individuals have a significantly higher incidence of accidents, especially repeated ones, than responsible and normally adjusted individuals.

Early exposure to injury, violence, domestic strife, over-authoritative parents or parent figures or the loss of parents are prominent elements in the histories of accident repeaters; these factors, among others, are believed to contribute to the development of a high degree of susceptibility to accidents.

Accidents due to aggressive behavior are nearly twice as frequent in irresponsible-maladjusted individuals (23.0%) as in normally adjusted-responsible individuals (13.9%).

Accidents are most likely to occur when the individual is under great mental, emotional, physical or physiological stress or strain.

An accident is almost certain to occur in a young man, age twenty-one, having a maladjusted-irresponsible background, driving at high speed, under emotional strain on a congested highway during a holiday on a hot and humid summer day.

Some accident patients express feelings of anxiety, guilt and deserved punishment soon after injury, but retract or deny these feelings a day or so later.

Some patients appear to exhibit a tendency to have accidents on certain days of the week or month or during certain hours of the day. This tendency seems to be especially marked on days or hours that are of symbolic significance to the individual.

These observations tend to support the theory of others that psychological gain plays a role in some accidents and that some injuries may have symbolic significance to the individual.

Even a trivial injury may be an outward manifestation of an underlying emotional strain or conflict.

The patient who merely gets his wounds dressed and is otherwise ignored or neglected, is more likely to develop traumatic or compensation neurosis and is more likely to suffer another and perhaps a more serious accident.

CAUSE

No satisfactory theory of accident causation has been evolved as yet.

Only about ten per cent of the remaining problems can, at best, be affected through the control of environmental exposures (safety).

Benefits derived from safety measures have long since reached a plateau.

Eighty per cent of non-industrial accidents belong to one of six types: Falls, aggressive behavior, handling objects, foreign bodies, motor vehicles and stumbling.

The high accident frequency at the peak age of twenty to twenty-four is due primarily to four types of accidents: aggressive behavior, motor vehicles, handling objects and foreign bodies in the eyes.

In children, the high incidence of accidents at the peak age five to nine years, is due primarily to motor vehicles, stepping on objects and aggressive behavior.

Falls are the most frequent cause of non-industrial accidents at all ages except between twenty and forty when aggressive behavior is the chief cause of accidents.

In males, aggressive behavior is the chief cause of non-industrial accidents (19.5%) especially at the ages of fifteen to thirty-nine and sixty to sixty-four and is only slightly more frequent than falls, which account for 18.7% of the accidents.

Accidents often occur where no tangible hazard can be demonstrated. Nearly all the causative factors of accidents ultimately relate to the **human factor.**

Some patients with multiple accidents always are inclined to injure the same part of the body, whether by burning, cutting or fracturing, and still others show a tendency towards accidents of a specific type, such as automobile accidents. (Dunbar)

Forty per cent of patients with recurrent accidents worked in fields unsuitable for their emotional constitution. (Csillag and Hedri)

FORTUITY

Not more than fifteen per cent of the total of all accidents arise purely from circumstances of fortuity.

FREQUENCY

Annual numbers of accidents in the U.S.A.:
95,000 killed
400,000 permanently injured
10,000,000 injured, with one or more days of disability
$10,000,000,000 direct and indirect expenditures

DAILY NUMBERS OF ACCIDENTS

260 killed
26,000 injured, with one or more days of disability.
One-fifth of the total population are directly or indirectly affected by accidents annually.
The accident rate at the age of twenty to twenty-four, in both the industrial and the non-industrial series, is 2.5 times higher than at the age of forty to forty-four, four times higher than at the age of fifty to fifty-four and nine times higher than at the age of sixty to sixty-four.

BODY AREA

More than seventy per cent of non-industrial injuries are concentrated in a relatively small area of the body;—the upper extremities, the head and the neck.

The upper extremities are most frequently injured in accidents. In children, the head and neck are most frequently injured. Injuries to the lower extremities are relatively more frequent in females and in older persons.

Injuries to the chest are relatively more frequent in older persons and injuries to the back in females of all ages, etc.

The fingers, the eyes and the hands are among the five most important sites of injury in both industrial and non-industrial accidents. Together

they account for 30.2% of the non-industrial and 47.9% of the industrial ones.
In children under the age of ten years, the three most frequent sites of injury are the face (18.5%) the scalp (10.7%) and the mouth (7.0%).
A comparative study of the number of injuries per accident and of the number of anatomical units involved in each accident shows that: there are more of these in non-industrial than in industrial accidents; more in older than in younger persons; more in females than in males and more in the maladjusted-irresponsible group than in the normally adjusted.

EPIDEMICS OF ACCIDENTS

Accidents are known to occur in epidemic form in industrial establishments as well as during holidays and week-ends.

THE ACCIDENT SYNDROME

The ability to diagnose the accident syndrome depends on an intimate knowledge of predisposing factors, environmental hazards, known trigger mechanisms and a past history of the behavior pattern of the individual when confronted with a sudden decision or danger.

Familiarity with the more important accident factors and the prevailing combinations of factors should enable the clinician to evaluate the probability of an accident in any given set of circumstances or individuals.

Viewing accidents as a disease syndrome may serve to reorient the physician to a more serious consideration of the causes, prevention and clinical treatment of accidents per se, and away from the almost exclusive preoccupation with only one of the sequelae or surface manifestations of accidents—the injury.

In the case of minor injuries, the physician-patient relationship is often that of an annoyed physician and an apologetic patient. A golden opportunity for psychological diagnosis and preventive efforts is thus unrecognized while the patient is cheerfully revealing his maladjustments to the nurse or attendant.

All the foregoing major findings and conclusions chiefly stem from the content of this book. Although no attempt has been made to indicate the pages within the body of the book leading to a particular conclusion, basis for all statements may be found within the text and foremostly within that long chapter entitled, "Charts and Tables." The hope is that a reading of these conclusions may provide impetus to investigate the more extensive data here presented in epitomization.

COMMENT ON CONCLUSIONS

The reduction of major findings and conclusions to epitomizing statements is sometimes insufficient to the exposition of these major findings and conclusions. Hence, it appears desirable briefly to extend a few of these items:

Age

In the total nineteen-year non-industrial series, 1930-1948, the incidence of accidents decreased from 8.6% in the age group four-nine to 7.3% in the age group ten-fourteen, then increased to a peak of 14.8% in the age group twenty-twenty-four after which the accidents decreased steadily until at age sixty-sixty-four they were only 1.8% of the total.

The industrial accident frequency increased from 9.2% in the age groups fifteen-nineteen to a peak of eighteen per cent in the age group twenty-twenty-four, then decreased steadily until, at the age of sixty-sixty-four they were only 2.1% of the total.

Studies by yearly age groups showed the highest incidence of accidents at the ages of twenty-one and twenty-two. Precipitous increments in percentage began at age seventeen, continued to the peak, then decreased with each year of age until twenty-eight. This mountainous hump in the percentage of accidents from ages seventeen to twenty-eight years appears to be real and significant. Certainly activities aimed at prevention should be directed in large part at persons in these age groups.

Among children, under fifteen years, the first and thirteenth years showed low percentages of accidents, while those aged two, four and eight years had relatively high percentages of accidents. In studies by five-year age groups, those ten-fourteen years old had the lowest percentage of accidents and less than any other five-year group under the age of forty-forty-four years.

There is a significant difference between the age distribution of patients with single accidents and those with multiple or repeated accidents. In patients with single accidents, the age distribution follows the pattern of distribution of the total sample, reaching a peak at the age of twenty-twenty-four; while in patients with multiple accidents the peak incidence is reached at the very early age of five-nine years.

The early age-peak in patients with multiple accidents is due primarily to the patients of the maladjusted and irresponsible group.

The high incidence of accidents in young persons is demonstrated by the finding that seventy per cent of accidents in the non-industrial series occurred before the age of thirty-five and nearly fifty per cent before the age of twenty-five.

Sex

The present studies indicate that males have a true and significantly higher incidence of accidents than females. All the non-industrial series revealed a consistent two to one ratio of accidents in males as compared to females. The same two to one ratio was obtained among patients with single accidents and patients with multiple or repeated accidents. The true ratio of male to female non-industrial accidents per unit time of exposure is probably much higher than the indicated two to one ratio, since approximately seventy per cent of the women and only thirty per cent of the men had a daily sixteen-hour exposure to non-industrial accidents.

In the industrial series, women averaged only 10.6% of the accidents and 11.8% of the patients during the nineteen-year period of 1930-1948. The ratio of male to female industrial accidents varied little from year to year except that during the depression years, 1930-1933, women contributed only about seven per cent of the industrial accidents, and during the war years, fourteen per cent.

Considering that during the period of study, an average of more than two men were employed in industry for each woman, the ratio of male to female industrial accidents at the observed rate of incidence would have been in the proportion of approximately two to one, if both sexes had been employed in equal numerical strength. Thus, there is an indicated two to one ratio of male to female accident potential in industrial as well as in non-industrial pursuits.

The greater susceptibility to accidents of the male is also demonstrated by a comparative study of repeated or multiple accidents. In the industrial series, 14.3% of the male patients and 4.8% of the female patients had two or more accidents annually during the entire nineteen-year period, 1930 through 1948, or a male to female accident ratio of three to one. The total number of accidents sustained by the multiple-accident patients, over the nineteen-year period of study, averaged 27.8% for the males and 9.7% for the females. A comparative study of patients with three or more accidents per annum is even more instructive, with regard to the degrees of susceptibility of both sexes. In the industrial group, 2.9% of the male patients and only 0.4% of the female patients averaged three or more accidents per annum. In the non-industrial series there was a fairly consistent two to one male to female ratio in the groups with two, three and four or more accidents per patient. Neither the industrial series nor the non-industrial ones showed any female patients with more than four accidents per annum, whereas among the males there were many patients with ten or more accidents in a single year.

A study of the non-industrial series by age and sex in single and in five-year age groups revealed that males had a higher incidence of accidents at every age level and every year of life, except the first. The difference in the accident rate of males and females narrows steadily and significantly at the extremes of life, especially at the ages of birth to four and at the age of sixty and older.

Age and Sex Distribution in Illness Compared to Accidents

The age and sex distribution of three thousand consecutive cases of illness from all causes, treated in 1947-1948, were analyzed as a control study. A comparison of the sex distribution of the patients showed that in contrast to the unequal distribution of the sexes in the accident series, both sexes are nearly equally represented at every age level of the illness groups; while the age distribution of the illness patients was practically identical with that of the accident patients.

The incidence of illness was found to decrease sharply from a relatively high rate of 12.7% in infants and children of the age birth to four years to a low rate of 3.5% at the age of ten-fourteen. The rate of illness then rose precipitously to a peak of 19.4% at the age of twenty-twenty-four, after which it decreased steadily with increment in age. During the peak ages of illness, ages birth to four and twenty-twenty-four, there was a relatively higher percentage of illness than accidents.

The equal distribution of the sexes in the illness groups lends added significance to the unequal distribution of the sexes in the accident series. Furthermore, this evidence reduces the likelihood that some selective factor other than accident tendency was responsible for the age and sex distribution of the accident patients. The nearly identical age distribution of the illness and accident groups also tends to support the theory that a common factor or factors predisposes individuals to illness and accidents at certain ages and increases their resistance to both at other ages. The "choice" of illness or accidents presumably depends on genetic endowment, environmental determinants and/or psychological needs or factors. A sharp division was sometimes seen between the "choice" of injury or illness in that many patients, including entire family groups, over a period of many years had accidents and virtually no illnesses, and others with an assorted variety of illness had no accidents. It would seem that "proneness" to accidents like "proneness" or susceptibility to illness represents a problem in general morbidity.

Multiple or Repeated Accidents

Numerous studies of the frequency distribution of accidents have indicated with monotonous regularity that most accidents occur in a relatively small group of individuals. This finding furnished the statistical basis upon which the psychological theory of "accident-proneness" was founded.

In twenty-five years of experience, the author has been unable to confirm the above observation. Although patients with repeated or multiple accidents were seen frequently, rarely were these found to continue in their accident habit when the period of observation was more than three years. Most of the accidents were found to be solitary experiences of many individuals, while the patients with repeated accidents were relatively few and these contributed only a moderate proportion of the total.

The analyzed series of industrial and non-industrial accidents were found to support the earlier clinical observations. The data showed that most of the accidents were due to large numbers of individuals with single accidents and not to a small group of highly "accident-prone" persons or accident repeaters. Although some patients had more accidents than others, those with multiple accidents accounted for less than thirty per cent of the total. This was a constant finding in both male and female for nearly every year of the nineteen-year period of study of the industrial series, and was equally true for both male and female in Groups A and B of the non-industrial series. The frequency distribution of the single and multiple accident patients was found to be approximately the same whether one, two, three, six, eleven or nineteen years were used as the unit of time for measuring accident experience.

The industrial series showed an average of 72.2% single accidents and 27.8% multiple accidents among men; and 90.3% single accidents and 9.7% multiple accidents among women. When the patients with single or multiple accidents were studied instead of their accidents, the disproportion in the distribution was even greater. Of the male industrial patients, only 14.3% had multiple accidents; while in females only 4.8% had multiples ones.

In the non-industrial series of *cases,* males and females combined averaged 16.3% multiple accidents, while the non-industrial *patients,* averaged only 7.8% multiple accidents. These data refer to industrial accidents as measured by yearly experience, and to non-industrial accidents as measured over the entire nineteen-year period, 1930 to 1948.

From another study it was learned that the number of patients treated for accidents during every year of a six-year period was extremely small. In the period 1936-1941, only 0.1% of the male industrial patients, were treated in each of these years. Of the remaining patients, 0.7% were treated in five consecutive years, 2.1% in four consecutive years and 7.1% in three consecutive years. The vast majority of the patients who were treated for repeated accidents were seen in only one year of the six-year period, and a slightly smaller percentage in two consecutive years. Specifically, 46.7% of the patients had multiple accidents during any one year of the six-year period; while 43.3% were treated for either single or multiple accidents in two consecutive years. With minor variations, the same results were obtained when the accident experience of these patients was studied for any two or more years of the six-year period instead of consecutive years.

Comparable results were also obtained when multiple accidents alone were considered. In the three three-year periods, 1935-1937, 1942-1944 and 1946-1948, an average of only 13.4% of the patients with multiple industrial accidents in one year incurred them also in any one of the other two years; multiple accidents in any two consecutive years were found in 9.9% of the patients and 4.2% of the patients incurred multiple accidents during the first and third years of the respective periods of study. Only about 0.5% of the patients had multiple accidents during every year of any three-year period. A similar survey of male non-industrial patients produced identical results. Multiple accidents among female non-industrial patients were so rare that the series was not used in this study.

In the patients with single or infrequent accidents, as in the total accident population, the highest incidence was reached at the age of twenty through twenty-four; while in the patients with multiple accidents, the highest incidence was reached at the age of five through nine.

The concept of accident proneness as a fixed personality factor which compels or generates accidental injury throughout life or long periods of time is incompatible with these findings.

The Incidence of Accidents in Irresponsible and Maladjusted Individuals

In their studies of the personality structure of patients with fractures, Dunbar *et al.*, have pointed to certain personality traits which, although not pathognomonic, were encountered with a degree of frequency which they considered highly significant. Among the more frequently encountered character traits were sexual and other forms of irresponsibility, as well as vocational and various other types of maladjustments.

The author suspected that those of his non-industrial patients who failed to honor their financial obligations and whose records were ultimately placed in an uncollectable file, possessed characteristics of irresponsibility and maladjustment described by Dunbar *et al.* The accident experience of this group of patients, designated as Group B, was studied, therefore, apart from all the other non-industrial accident patients who were designated as Group A.

A comparative study of the frequency of repeated or multiple accidents in the normally adjusted Group A and in the irresponsible and maladjusted Group B showed that of all the accidents in Group B, 21.5% were multiple ones, as against 13.9% in Group A—an increase of fifty-four per cent in the frequency of multiple accidents in Group B over A. Nearly identical results were obtained when the numbers of patients with multiple accidents were compared instead of their accidents. The difference in the accident frequency of Groups A and B was found to grow in almost geometric proportion when the number of accidents per person increased from two to three or four and more. Thus, in patients with two accidents each, the excess accident frequency in Group B over A was only twelve per cent; in patients with three accidents each, the excess was one hundred and fifteen per cent; while in patients with four or more accidents each, the excess of accidents in Group B over A was four hundred and fifty-five per cent.

Somewhat higher differences were obtained when the patients of the two groups were compared instead of their accidents.

The comparative frequency of multiple or repeated accidents in Groups A and B at different ages, was chiefly studied as the sum of each of four different periods: 1930-1941, 1942-1944, 1945 and 1946-1948, and again as the total of the entire 1930-1948 period. The results obtained from both of these studies show a high degree of correlation.

The higher incidence of accidents in the maladjusted and irresponsible individuals (Group B) was especially marked in the young patients under the age of twenty-five. Of all the multiple accidents in Group B, 85.2% occurred before the age of thirty-five and 71.5% before the age of twenty-five; while in Group A, only sixty per cent of the multiple accidents occurred before the age of thirty-five and only 44.5% before the age of twenty-five. Counting all the accidents, single as well as multiple, 79.2% of the accidents in Group B and 65.8% of those in Group A occurred in the first half-span of life; while in females of Group B nearly eighty-three per cent occurred during this period of time.

The difference in the accident frequency of Groups A and B was especially prominent in their children. The children of the maladjusted and irresponsible homes (Group B) were found to have a significantly higher incidence of accidents than the children of the normally adjusted patients (Group A). In Group B, 30.7% of all the accidents occurred before the age of fifteen, while in Group A, only 21.6% of the accidents occurred before this age. The difference was even greater when the multiple or repeated accidents of the two groups were compared. In Group B, 46.2% of the multiple accidents occurred before the age of fifteen; while in Group A, only twenty-seven per cent occurred before the same age.

The difference in the age distribution of the accidents in Groups A and B was also highly significant. In Group A, the incidence of accidents decreased steadily from early childhood to the age of ten through fourteen years, while in Group B, there was an increase in accident rate at the age of five through nine before the usual decline at the age of ten through fourteen. The contrast in the age distribution of the patients with multiple or repeated accidents in Groups A and B was most remarkable. In Group A the incidence of multiple accidents remained at a relatively low and fairly even level of distribution of eight to nine per cent throughout the greater part of life, or up to the age of fifty, when they began to decrease with further increment in age. In Group B, on the other hand, multiple accidents rose precipitously to a high peak of twenty to twenty-one per cent at the very young age of five through nine and then decreased steadily with increment in age. In Group A, the age distribution of young patients with multiple accidents was only slightly above the normal age distribution of the general population of Cincinnati (U. S. Census 1930 and 1940); while in Group B, the age distribution of the patients with multiple accidents under the age of twenty-five was significantly higher than either in Group A or in the general population.

In the total series of single and multiple accidents of Groups A and B combined, the accident frequency rate increased at the age of five through nine; decreased to a low at the age of ten through fourteen; rose to a peak at the age of twenty through twenty-four and then decreased steadily with increment in age. In the females of both Groups A and B and in all the patients of Group A, the accident frequency continued to decline through the age of five through nine to reach the common low at the age of ten through fourteen. Otherwise the curve of age distribution was the same as in the total series.

The above studies indicate that persons belonging to maladjusted and irresponsible families tend to have a significantly higher incidence of accidents, solitary as well as multiple ones, than those not so designated. This group (B) of patients is especially noted for the very high rate of accidents among their children, particularly during the age of five through nine years, an age when the over-all accident rate is otherwise very low. At the peak of accident frequency, age twenty through twenty-four, the incidence of accidents in Group B was 16.4% compared to 14.1% in Group A.

From the foregoing it is apparent that a small percentage of a given population can account for most of the accidents on the basis of youth alone or the presence in such a population of an undue number of irresponsible and maladjusted individuals. The presence of both of these factors at one and the same time accentuates the unequal distribution of the accidents.

An important group has thus been identified in the general population, the irresponsible and maladjusted group that has a high frequency of accidents and apparently contributes a disproportionate share to the total number of accidents. This high-accident-frequency group has been further identified with regard to the ages at which most of the accidents occur. In contrast to other methods of study the above described groups of "accident-prone" individuals are easily recognizable by means of a good clinical history.

The Incidence of Accidents in Relation to the Annual Cycle

Early in the course of an active industrial medical practice was noted a seasonal fluctuation in the frequency of injuries by accident. Year after year, over a period of more than twenty years, the same pattern of a relatively high frequency of accidents during the summer months and a much lower incidence during the winter months has repeated itself. An analysis of the monthly variations in frequency of large series of industrial and non-industrial accidents confirmed these clinical observations and revealed, in addition, a cyclical pattern of distribution.

Incidence by Months

Both the industrial and the non-industrial series show a low incidence of accidents in February and a peak in August. In the non-industrial series there is a steady rise in the percentage of total accidents from a low of 6.2% in February to a high of 10.8% in August, followed by a steady decline to February. The total industrial series shows an equally low percentage of accidents in February of 6.9% and a high in August of 9.6%. The rise and fall of the monthly incidence of the industrial accidents is not as precipitous as the monthly incidence of the non-industrial accidents; the trend, however, is similar. The summer peak of the industrial accidents extended over the four-month period, June-September, and in the non-industrial series over a three-month period, June-August.

The monthly distribution of the accidents is similar in both male and female.

Analysis of the male non-industrial series disclosed a steady rise in the frequency of the accidents from a low of six per cent during the month of February to a high of eleven per cent in June. The frequency rate declined slightly in July and August, then more rapidly until it reached a low in February. There is nearly one-hundred per cent range of difference between the low accident rate of February and the high accident rate of June. The rates of rise and fall in accident frequency to and from the summer peaks are nearly equal.

In the broad fifteen-year age groups, the male non-industrial series shows that with increment in age there is a steady decline in the percentage of summer injuries, as well as in the range of difference between the low accident rate of winter and the high rate of summer. In boys under fifteen years of age, the range of difference between the summer high and the winter low is about two hundred and thirty per cent while in men past forty-five, the range of difference is only about fifty per cent. Boys under fifteen years of age have the highest incidence of accidents in July, the hottest month of the year in Cincinnati, and show a more perfect cyclical pattern of distribution than any other age group. With increment in age, the annual accident frequency curve steadily flattens and the peak shifts from June in the age group fifteen through twenty-nine, to July and August in the age group thirty through forty-four and to August in the age group forty-five and older.

The female non-industrial accidents of all age groups reach a peak frequency in August. This is reflected in a sharp one month peak in the female as compared to a blunt three-month peak (June-August) in the male. The range of difference between the highest monthly incidence and the lowest is nearly identical in both male and female non-industrial accidents. In the females, as in males, both the percentage of summer injuries and the range of difference between the summer high and the winter low decrease steadily with increment in age.

The low incidence of accidents in February of six to seven per cent is identical for both sexes and for every age group. The three summer months account for thirty-two per cent (or one third) of all the accidents in both sexes. In the males the percentage of summer accidents decreased steadily from thirty-nine per cent in boys under fifteen years of age, to twenty-eight per cent in men past forty-five. In females, the precentage of summer injuries decreased steadily from thirty-five per cent in the youngest group to twenty-six per cent in the oldest.

Seasonal Incidence of Accidents

A comparison of the seasonal distribution of the industrial and non-industrial accidents, male and female combined, showed a remarkable resemblance in all major respects. In both series, in the order of the diminishing frequency of accidents, summer is followed by fall, spring and winter.

Both industrial and non-industrial accidents show comparable decreases in the frequency of summer accidents with increment in age. The non-industrial accidents show a wider range of difference between the summer high and the winter low than the industrial accidents. In the non-industrial group, thirty-two per cent of the accidents occurred in the summer months and 20.3% in the winter months; while in the industrial series, 29.5% occurred in the summer and 22.2% in the winter. The percentage of fall injuries with 25.5% and spring injuries with 22.5% was nearly identical for both groups.

A major difference between the industrial and the non-industrial series was found in the steady increase with increment in age, of winter accidents in the non-industrial group and of autumn accidents in the industrial group.

To determine the effect of increased summer activity on the seasonal incidence of accidents, the writer studied the ratio of school-hour accidents, 8:00 a.m. to 3:00 p.m., to non-school-hour accidents in children of school age (6 to 15). Since at least five of the eight school hours are spent in the classroom, one would expect increases in the ratio of school-hour accidents during the summer when the children are out of school and are given to the more hazardous activity of outdoor play. Surprisingly, the ratio of school-hour to non-school-hour accidents remained unchanged during summer, fall and winter. In the spring a significant increase was noted in the ratio of non-school-hour accidents.

The industrial series provides further evidence that the observed differences in the frequencies of summer and winter accidents are not necessarily due to differences in levels of industrial activity. One series of industrial accidents studied occurred during the war years, 1942-1944. These years were characterized by a sustained all-year around high level of industrial activity. Yet the seasonal frequency of the accidents fluctuated significantly in the described manner and resembles closely the seasonal frequency distribution of the non-industrial series.

The Incidence of Accidents in Relation to the Diurnal Cycle

Investigating a large controlled series of industrial accidents in England, Vernon found that the hours of 10:00 a.m. and 3:00 p.m. have the highest rate of accidents in the 8:00 a.m. to 5:00 p.m. day shift. In a study of night shift accidents, Osborne and Vernon found that most of these accidents occurred during the first few hours of work and relatively few during the last hours. The hourly accident rate declined steadily as the night progressed towards the morning and was at a minimum during the last one-and-a-half hours of work. The accident frequency was generally lower during the night shift than during the day.

The frequently reported high frequency of industrial accidents during the housr of 10:00 a.m. and 3:00 p.m. in day workers and during the early evening hours in night workers are in full agreement with the author's own clinical experience and studies.

Analysis of the hourly distribution of the industrial accidents showed a steady increase in accident frequency during the first two hours of work of both the morning and afternoon shifts, culminating in a peak during the third hour, and then dropping in a like manner during the fourth or last hour of each half shift. The noon hour was marked by a very low incidence of accidents, thereby accentuating the double peak for the total work period. All of the industrial samples showed identical patterns of the hourly distribution of accidents.

The men workers had the same frequency of accidents during the morning half of the day shift as during the afternoon, while the women workers had a higher frequency during the morning hours. The hourly distribution of the accidents in the women workers differed somewhat from the standard pattern of distribution in that the accident frequency remained at a relatively low and even level during the last three hours of the afternoon shift.

During the morning hours, the accident frequency of the male workers increased from 7.6% during the hour of 8:00 a.m. to 16.7% during the hour of 10:00 a.m.; while in women workers, it increased during the same hours from 9.7% to 19.3%. In the afternoon hours, the male accidents increased from 10.1% during the hour of 1:00 p.m. to 15.5% during the hour of 3:00 p.m.; while in women, the accident frequency increased from 9.2% during the first hour to 11.1% during the second hour. This level of accident frequency was maintained during the remaining hours of the afternoon.

Of the industrial accidents, both male and female, 84.5% occurred during the prevailing workday hours of 8:00 a.m. to 5:00 p.m. and 13.5% during the remaining fifteen hours of the diurnal cycle. In the male workers, 47.2% of the accidents occurred during the morning and an equal number, or 47.4% occurred during the afternoon, while in the female workers 49.8% of the accidents occurred during the morning and only forty-three per cent during the afternoon. During the noon hour the women workers had a somewhat higher accident frequency than the men, namely 7.2% for women against 5.4% for men. When studied by twelve hour periods, 90.4% of the accidents to men occurred in the period from 6:00 a.m. to 6:00 p.m., 42.2% in the six hours before noon and 48.2% in the six hours after noon. In women, a somewhat different distribution was obtained—92.5% of the accidents occurred during the twelve hour period with an equal division of 46.3% during each of the six hour periods before and after noon.

The hourly frequency rate of the 15.5% of the indstrial accidents which occurred during the fifteen hour period of 5:00 p.m. to 8:00 a.m. decreased steadily throughout the night hours; except that there

MAJOR FINDINGS AND CONCLUSIONS

were low grade peaks during the hours of 8:00 p.m., 10:00 to 11:00 p.m. and during the hour of 4:00 a.m. in women. The hour of lowest accident frequency for the entire twenty-four hour period was 5:00 a.m. This was true for all the samples studied, both industrial and non-industrial. It may be of interest to note that the diurnal distribution of accidents observed in the present uncontrolled group of industrial cases corresponds closely to that found by Osborne and Vernon (60) in their much larger and well controlled series.

Analysis of the *industrial* patients by five-year age groups showed that while the over-all accident rate varied with age, the relative hourly frequency did not and was nearly identical for all age groups studied.

A further breakdown of the hour of accident occurrence into fifteen minute periods revealed a tendency to report the accident in terms of integrated hours and to a lesser extent, in half and quarter hours. About fifty per cent of the accidents were reported to have occurred on the hour, another twenty-five per cent on the half-hour and the remaining twenty-five per cent were divided about equally between the quarter hours. An exception to this rule was the hour of 8:00 a.m. when more accidents were reported on the half-hour.

Analysis of the hourly frequency of the non-industrial accidents revealed a diurnal cyclical pattern of distribution in both the male and female series. In both sexes the hourly frequency of the non-industrial accidents increased steadily with a low at 5:00 a.m. to a peak at 3:00 to 5:00 p.m. and then declined again to the low frequency of the early morning hours.

The male non-industrial patients showed peak frequencies during the hours of 10:00 a.m., 3:00 p.m., 5:00 p.m., 8:00 p.m. and 2:00 a.m.; and the female patients showed similar peaks during the hours of 6:00 a.m., 8:00 a.m., 11:00 a.m., 5:00 p.m., 8:00 p.m. and 2:00 a.m. The male and female hourly accident frequencies tend to follow parallel courses and have identical peaks at certain hours. A comparison with the industrial series showed that the diurnal hours of high accident frequency were identical in the males of both the industrial and non-industrial series. The female accidents were too few for the required multiple breakdowns to permit significant correlations.

A study of the hourly frequency of *non-industrial* accidents in three broad age groups showed that each age has a diurnal accident frequency of its own. In children of both sexes under the age of fifteen years, most of the accidents occurred between the hours of 3:00 p.m. and 8:00 p.m. and were at peak frequency during the hours of 3:00 p.m. for boys and 5:00 p.m. for girls. The frequency of the accidents as well as the range of increase during the peak hours was greater in this age group than in any other.

In the age group fifteen to thirty-nine, the hour of 10:00 p.m. had the highest incidence of accidents in both males and females. The period of high accident frequency in this age group extended over more hours than either in the younger or the older age groups. The accident frequency in the age group fifteen to thirty-nine increased from 5:00 a.m. to 3:00 p.m. and again from 6:00 p.m. to 10:00 p.m. The male and female hourly frequency curves coincided more closely in the age group fifteen to thirty-nine than in either the younger or the older age groups.

In the age group forty and older, there was a relatively high accident frequency during the hour of 9:00 a.m. and the highest rate was between the hours of 3:00 p.m. and 6:00 p.m. Both the male and the female hourly distributions of accidents in this age group of forty and over are less differentiated than in both younger age groups; yet the same general cyclical trend is discernible even here.

The hourly distribution of the non-industrial accidents in the different age groups was studied for purposes of comparison with the industrial series. In the older age groups of both series the hours of 10:00 to 11:00 p.m. are peak hours for accidents. The male and female distributions are more closely correlated in this age group than in any of the others.

A study of the median hour of peak accident frequency showed that the hour of 4:00 p.m. was the median peak hour for accidents in the age group under fifteen years. Past the age of fifteen years, the median peak hour for accidents shifted steadily with increment in age from 6:00 p.m. at the ages of fifteen to thirty-nine; to 5:00 p.m. at the ages of thirty to forty-four; 4:00 p.m. at the ages of forty-five to fifty-nine and 3:00 p.m. at the ages of sixty and older. The median diurnal peak hour for accidents was thus observed to shift with increment in age from the early evening hours toward the early afternoon hours.

With increment in age there was also observed a flattening of the diurnal accident frequency curve.

It may be noted that 3:00 p.m. to 5:00 p.m. were the hours of highest accident frequency in children under fifteen years and in adults over forty; while in young adults ages fifteen to thirty-nine, 10:00 p.m. to 11:00 p.m. were the hours of highest accident frequency.

In both male and female, seventy per cent of the non-industrial accidents occurred between noon and midnight and these were equally divided between the hours of noon and 6:00 p.m. and between 6:00 p.m. and midnight. When the prevailing workday hours of 8:00 a.m. and 5:00 p.m. were considered, it was found that forty-two per cent of both the male and female non-industrial accidents occurred between these workday hours and fifty-eight per cent between the hours of 5:00 p.m. and 8:00 a.m. This identical per cent distribution of the non-industrial accidents in both sexes is interesting in view of the differences in the rates and types of exposure of male and female.

A cyclical pattern of hourly distribution of accidents is discernible in the industrial accident series and is unmistakable in the non-industrial series. These studies suggest a diurnal cycle in which the highest incidence of accidents is during the hours of 3:00 p.m. to 5:00 p.m. and the lowest at 5:00 a.m.

Hourly Distribution of Repeated Accidents

In those cases with a given history of three or more accidents each, the hours of occurence of the repeated accident were identical in more than half of the patients. In the industrial patients 74.4% of these multiple accidents occurred during identical hours, 14.4% in nearly identical hours and only 11.2% in unidentical hours. In the non-industrial group, 54.5% of the multiple accidents occurred during identical hours and the others in nearly identical hours. None of these accidents occurred in widely separated hours of the day. This was found to hold true for both male and female.

In the patients with a recorded history of only two accidents each, a much smaller percentage of the accidents occurred during identical hours, namely: 26.3% of the industrial accidents and 10.3% of the non-industrial accidents.

CHAPTER THREE

CONCEPTS OF ACCIDENT CAUSATION

Search for a common denominator in the many theories of accident causation becomes a rugged task. There are no anlagen serving to bring about unification. This is not expectable nor is it desirable that simplification be sought in the delineation of the multipotent factors that contribute to the genesis of accidents. The array of concepts here to be epitomized introduces complexity rather than homogeneity.

1. INTRODUCTION AND HISTORY

The study of accidents as an organized body of knowledge largely is the product of the present century. The earliest studies concerned themselves primarily with the treatment of injuries due to accidents. With the advent of the factory system, the railroad, the automobile, the insurance carrier and the workmen's compensation laws, there developed an interest in causative factors and preventive measures.

An imposing number of research studies by a host of investigators resulted. Yet, considering the seriousness of the problem and the staggering cost of accidents in terms of human and financial resources, the sum total of basic research dealing with accidents is surprisingly meager and wanting.

During the first three decades of this century, when "carelessness" was the generally accepted "cause" of most accidents, "safety" appeared to be the logical answer to the problem. The safety movement was greatly encouraged and stimulated by startling initial results. Soon a point of diminishing returns was reached and most workers in the field are now in agreement that results obtainable from such safety measures as guards, goggles, slogans, campaigns, education, etc., and the elimination of physical hazards, have reached a plateau and little further progress can be expected from this avenue of approach.

Much useful information became available as a result of the study of hazards (51, 60, 68, 69, 71) and there is general agreement that the elimination of environmental hazards remains, at the present, one of the most fruitful means of checking the annual accident toll. Most accidents, however, occur in or about the home where the environmental hazards are of relatively low degree and difficult to control (51, 71). Even in industry accidents often occur where no tangible hazards can be demonstrated. It was further discovered that, more often than not, the hazard, as well as the accident, is a product of human failings such as haste, distraction, preoccupation or faulty judgment. It has also been demonstrated that human failings are, in turn, frequently related to states of emotional strain or conflict in which elements of anxiety, anger, fear, frustration, hate, aggression and guilt play a vital role (1, 17, 42, 43, 50). Workers in the field, therefore, began to turn their attention to, and put greater emphasis upon, studies dealing with the relation of accidents to human behavior.

A new factor was thus added to the etiology of accidents—the personality factor—a hazard arising from within the individual or from the interaction of the human personality with its environment. These findings gave a new stimulus, as well as a new direction, to research in the field and a considerable part of the literature of the past twenty-five years deals with methods of detection and treatment of "accident-prone" individuals and with the psychodynamics of accidents and "accident-proneness."

The history of the concept of "accident-proneness" dates back to 1919 when Greenwood and Woods (29) and Greenwood and Yule (30) made their first thorough investigation of the distribution of accidents. Their findings and conclusions were later critically examined and extended by Newbold (46, 47). In a recent critical review of the subject, Arbous (7) stated that after a quarter of a century, the work of Greenwood *et al.* must still be regarded as almost complete summaries of our existing knowledge of this phenomenon. "In these studies, the reader will find the basic assumptions on which the concept of proneness depends, but also the essential warnings of the limitations of these same assumptions which have been unhappily disregarded."

Greenwood and Woods reported the results of an analysis of the accidents suffered by workers in the British munition factories during World War I. They made the then startling finding that mishaps are not evenly distributed among persons who are equally exposed to identical environmental hazards. They learned that some persons have significantly more accidents than others, and that a relatively small percentage of the population have most of the accidents. The shape of the resulting histogram suggested some regular features about it and implied an underlying principle which could be stated in some law of distribution.

In an effort to explain the observed unequal distribution of the accidents, Greenwood *et al.* examined three theoretical possibilities: (1) That the distribution was due to pure chance (in the same sense as the chance of drawing a given card from a well-shuffled deck of cards would be on an average once in every fifty-two times) and was governed by Poisson's law of distribution; (2) that the distribution was biased—although starting with an initial equal liability to accidents, those who sustain one accident by pure chance might thereby have their probability of having further accidents either increased or decreased, and (3) that the observed distribution was due to an unequal initial liability—some persons are inherently more liable to have accidents than others.

Greenwood's hypothesis of unequal initial liability to accidents was subsequently taken up by psychologists and by psychiatric investigators and, stimulated by a current wave of enthusiasm for mental health, psychosomatic medicine and analytical psychiatry, it has led to a rapid, overwhelming and uncritical acceptance of the psychological concept of accident-proneness as the cause of most accidents. The prevailing impression among lay and professional persons alike is that most accidents are due to a small fixed group of "accident-prone" individuals who are under a deep psychological necessity or cumpulsion to have accidents and that a solution of the accident problem depends on identification and treatment of these "accident-prone" individuals.

Farmer and Chambers (21) declare: "Previous statistical investigations have shown that industrial workers exposed to equal risks were unequal in their liability to sustain accidents, and that this unequal liability was a relatively stable phenomenon, manifesting itself in different periods of exposure and in different kinds of accidents. . . . . ."

The British Medical Research Council (69) corroborates the postulate that, under like conditions of exposure and environment, some people have more accidents than others. This difference in accident rate might be attributed to various causes, but scientific analysis has shown the special importance of the factor known as "accident-proneness" described as a fixed set of personal qualities which render certain individuals more likely to sustain accidents than others. "Study of a number of industrial groups, and also of several groups of transport drivers, has shown that there is a tendency for those who have an undue number of accidents in one period to have an undue number in all subsequent periods . . . . each hour of the day, each day of the week, each month of the year and each subsequent year."

The same attitude is echoed in the Transactions of the 35th National Safety Congress: "A relatively small number of employees account for the great majority of industrial injuries. . . . In fact, the elimination of the accident-proneness of these employees (eight per cent) would result in a forty-five per cent decrease in total minor injuries."

On the basis of epidemiological studies, clinical observations and thorough reviews of the mathematics of the original formulation of the unequal initial liability theory, various investigators have, in recent years, begun to challenge the concept of "accident-proneness" as currently formulated. Arbous (7) deplores the kind of conclusions which were made by subsequent investigators concerning Greenwood's results: "Almost all the literature published after these studies regards the existence of accident-proneness as an established fact and that it is a stable component of the personality which makes it worth our while attempting to predict and to use in practical accident prevention measures."

The original observations of Greenwood and Woods were made on a group of six hundred and forty-eight female munition workers over a thirteen-month period. It may be noted that two-thirds of the women had no accidents at all, another twenty per cent had one accident each and about six per cent had two accidents each. The more frequent accidents (five to three) were suffered by twenty-six women: whereas on the basis of chance distribution, only eight women should have had multiple accidents.

A second method used by Greenwood and Woods to study accident distribution was to compare the accident rate of groups of women in two successive periods. They found that a group of one hundred and thirty-six women without accidents at the beginning of the period of observation had a mean monthly accident rate of 0.16 over a five-month period, while sixty-two women with one or two accidents had a mean monthly frequency rate of 0.35 over the same period or more than twice as many.

The third method of studying accident frequency distribution consisted of comparing the coefficients of correlation between the number of accidents incurred in successive periods. The accident experience of four groups of women studied over two successive three-month periods showed a positive correlation ranging from 0.37 ± 0.12 to 0.72 ± 0.07. When the persons without accidents during the first three-month period were excluded, a lower correlation ranging from 0.18 ± 0.17 to 0.63 ± 0.09 was obtained. If the hypothesis of biased distribution was correct, reasoned Greenwood *et al.*, the correlation should have been closer when the accident-free persons were removed.

Greenwood and Woods warned that it does not follow from these studies that the distribution of accidents is never biased by previous accidents or that some accidents are never incurred by pure chance.

The most important factors that have helped in the development and acceptance of the concept of "accident-proneness" as a stable psychological phenomenon were the analytical studies reported by Dunbar (17), Menninger (42, 43), Rawson (50), Ackerman and Chidester (1) and others. Some of the evidence which has helped in the process may be summarized as follows:

Marbe (39) in 1926, was the first to call the tendency towards multiple accidents the "accident habit." He provided statistical evidence that the probability for having accidents is greater for the person who has had previous accidents. He also suggested that the personality factor has more significance than the type of occupation in determining accident frequency.

"Accident-proneness," say Hildebrandt and Ross (33), is due to individual personal qualities such as hereditary taint, unsatisfied desires, the type of work, frequent change of work, a negative attitude to the job, unfavorable social conditions, depression and a biased outlook in general. Accidents may result from a state of depression, lack of inhibition, intoxication, etc. The rate of reaction and ability to adjust are not as important factors in "accident-proneness' as has usually been assumed. States of nervous exhaustion are more common among "accident-prone" individuals. Diseases are more common. Constitutional debility is not a factor; some of those most prone to accident are strongly-built husky individuals.

Heyman (32) asserts that technical factors are of less significance than the human element. "Accident-proneness" or predisposition is the determining factor. Dunbar (17) states that her evidence and the evidence of insurance companies suggests that in at least eighty per cent of accidents, the personality of the injured person was probably more responsible than machinery or training.

" 'Accident-prone' individuals are 'accident-prone' in any occupation," says Rawson (50). The National Research Council (70) reported a study of four large industrial concerns employing fourteen hundred drivers of trucks and commercial cars. One of the firms shifted the men with the highest accident rates to other jobs. In less than four years, this firm reduced its annual accident rate by four-fifths, but the men shifted to non-driving jobs began to have accidents in the plant or at home, instead of traffic accidents. They also found that the majority of accidents were the fault of the driver rather than the weather conditions, equipment or any other factors.

Greenwood and Woods (29) in a study of eight hundred and ninety-one omnibus drivers, and from the inspection of nearly six thousand additional insurance records, concluded that "accident-proneness" is a measurable quality.

This optimistic view of the measurability of "accident-proneness" has fallen short of realization. In a study to detect and treat "accident-prone" drivers, Johnson (35) concluded that the "best of all possible tests can do no more than sort the individuals into liability classes, such that the liability is the same for every individual within a specific class."

Despite a great deal of effort and the invention of a multitude of ingenious tests, the condition known as "accident-proneness" cannot be diagnosed at the present. A past history of multiple accidents does not necessarily indicate "accident-proneness," (1, 17, 47, 50) even if adequate allowance is made for unusual exposures, for hazards and for a variety of other factors. There is, furthermore, no agreement as to the exact combination of elapsed time between accidents, the number or frequency of accidents and the severity of the injuries which would classify an individual as "accident-prone."

The difficulty of detecting "accident-proneness" suggested to Adler (3) in 1934, the existence of an unknown "X" factor in the human personality which tended to cause the individual to subject himself to accident.

Farmer and Chambers (20) are credited with coining the term "accident-proneness." In defining "accident-proneness" they state: "The fact that one of the factors connected with accident liability has been found to be a peculiarity of the individual allows us to differentiate between 'accident-proneness' and 'accident liability.' Accident-proneness is a narrower term than accident liability and means a personal idiosyncrasy predisposing the individual who possesses it in a marked degree to a relatively high accident rate. Accident liability includes all the factors determining accident rate."

Vernon (60), one of the early and foremost investigators of the accident problem states: "The accident-proneness of various individuals is not a fixed quality, but is liable to be affected by any and every change in their bodily condition. This condition is influenced by external changes of environment as well as by internal changes of physical and mental health." Three years later, in 1939, the same author declared (61) that: "accident liability is influenced by many other personal qualities besides inherent accident-proneness. It depends on general health, age and experience, fatigue, etc. . . ."

Arbous (7) points out these conflicting views on the stability or instability of "accident-proneness" in order to illustrate the lack of precision in thinking on this subject: "It must be decided if accident-proneness is a stable or a variable attribute, a general or specific factor." He feels quite strongly that the term "accident-proneness" should be clearly defined before any practical use is made of it.

2. PSYCHODYNAMICS

Psychiatrists, beginning with Freud, have encountered individuals who have expressed or acted out self-destructive tendencies. That these expressions of subsconscious wishes have included accidents was presented by Menninger (42, 43) in 1936 after studying certain "accidents" which, on analysis, proved to have been unconsciously purposive. In many of the accidents studied, Menninger noted that although on the surface they appeared to be entirely fortuitous, they could be shown, on deeper analysis, to be aimed at partial or focal self-destruction. Menninger postulates that the patients sustained injuries which in certain accidents . . . "can be shown to fulfill so specifically unconscious tendencies of the victim that we are compelled to believe either that they represent the capitalization of some opportunity for self-destruction by the death instinct or else were in some obscure way brought about for this very purpose. . . ."

The ego refuses to accept responsibility for the self-destruction in purposive accidents and in some instances it shows great determination in making this evasion, says Menninger. The difference between fatal accidents and accidents in which only a part of the body is destroyed is assumed to be due to some failure of the death instinct for full participation.

The motive in accidents, as in other forms of self-destruction, such as suicide, self-mutilations and compulsive submission to surgery, says Menninger, includes the elements of aggression, punition and propitiation with death as the occasional but exceptional outcome. This observation leads the author to suspect that the principle of sacrifice is operative in accidents, so that in a sense the individual submits himself to the possibility or certainty of an accident in which he has at least a chance of escape rather than face certain destruction, which he fears, even though it may threaten him only in his conscience and imagination. The accident, according to Menninger, serves to neutralize the destructive impulses and is in the nature of a ransom which protects the ego against the fantasied death penalty.

In evaluating Menninger's theory, elaborated upon that of Freud, it should be noted that (a) the existence of a death instinct as the motive-force of self-destructive tendency is not universally or even generally accepted by analytical psychiatrists, and (b) Menninger did not conduct any quantitative studies and he offered the self-destructive theory of accident causation in a qualitative sense only as a possible cause of accidents in certain or selected cases.

Other dynamic psychiatrists emphasize the role of the super ego as a guilt producing mechanism. For such guilt, partial or total self-destruction offers assuagement. No primary death instinct is required in this hypothesis, since the sense of guilt arises out of conflicts between id drives and super ego standards.

The death instinct theory currently is less accepted. In its place now has been projected a quite contrary concept that the individual strives constantly for some form of adaptation and adequate integration; and where behavior becomes disturbed, it is an attempt on the part of the individual somehow to adapt to the new circumstances, even though inadequately. When the concept of the super ego which exacts punishment for guilt is counterpoised, it puts the destructive behavior of the individual in the area of defensive maneuvers rather than instinct per se. The importance of this is that it signifies that the individual is trying to adapt. While attempting to get rid of a discomfort, namely guilt, he is led into behavior which brings him into difficulty, but the tendency, the drive, is for adaptation and equilibrium.

While Menninger was presenting his evidence of the traumatophilic diathesis theory of Freud (25,26), Dunbar and her group were completing a five-year study of sixteen hundred fracture patients admitted to a general hospital, which lends additional psychiatric and some statistical support to this theory (17,18). Dunbar's work profoundly influenced the course of thinking on the accident problem over the past twenty years and remains the only large statistical study of the psychological aspect of "accident-proneness" to date.

Medical investigators already had accumulated a significant mass of evidence to confirm that bodily changes may be brought about by mental stimuli, by emotions, just as effectively as by bacteria and toxins, and that physiological changes accompanying emotion may disturb the function of any organ of the body. A substantial link between emotion and accidents, however, had not yet been proved. It was generally believed when their studies began, Dunbar points out, that the fracture group was the most "normal" of any group of patients under treatment and was, therefore, intended to be used as a control group. After studying the personalities of several groups of patients and their reactions to illness and treatment, Dunbar *et al.,* found marked similarities among the members of each group and equally marked differences among the several groups. As a result of these studies, Dunbar *et al.* became convinced that the "fracture patients as a group do not represent particularly 'normal' people."

Among other things, they found that forty per cent of the fracture group gave a history of accidents in the family and forty-six per cent gave a history of exposure to accidents in family or friend. This is more than three times higher than the percentage for family history of accidents found in any of the other groups studied. This finding suggested to the authors that there may be something in the general make-up of certain individuals which predisposes them to accidents and that this trait may run in families.

In observing patients with multiple accidents, Dunbar found that some of these patients were inclined to injure the same member, whether by burning, cutting or fracturing, and that still others showed a tendency toward accidents of a specific type, such as automobile accidents, etc.

Seventy per cent of the fracture patients supplied a childhood history of neurotic traits or habits of abnormal duration, such as nail-biting, eneuresis, truancy from school and a tendency to lie and steal; whereas only twenty per cent of the patients with cardiovascular diseases gave such a history. Sixty per cent of the fracture patients made a confession of guilt or resentment soon after the accident or endowed the accident with a purposive character of some sort, while only one per cent of the cardiac patients viewed their illness in this light.

The fracture patients were found to differ from the other groups studied by a low illness record, few operations, a high record of previous accidents, especially in childhood, a high percentage of childless marriages, small families and a high rate of divorce. Most of the "accident-prone" males showed a marked adventurous trend, sexual and other forms of irresponsibility and a tendency to live from day to day, to change jobs frequently and to have many and diversified jobs.

The behavior pattern of the fracture patients was found to differ from the others by an outward casualness about feelings and personal problems, a lack of planning, a tendency towards impulsive action and short-term goals. They displayed a striving for independent behavior or autonomy in their relationship with authoritarian figures, in contrast with a characteristic domination or submission found in the other illness groups. They were frequently boastful and liked to take long chances. They were relatively inarticulate and tended to act things out, rather than express them by words. The fracture group contained many eccentrics, but few psychoneurotics.

Dunbar believes that the sex of the individual per se is, not an important factor in the incidence of accidents; while the high accident frequency of youth is considered by her to be secondary to the short expectation of life of the "accident-prone." In Dunbar's fracture series, the incidence of accidents in males and females was nearly identical. At the same time she points out that female teenage drivers have a better accident record than males, and that fatal accidents of males and females are in the ratio of two to one. Dunbar makes clear that *conflicts* about sexuality do play a role in accident causation, thus females who have conflicts about menstruation, and their role as women tend to group their accidents around the time of their menstrual period. However, ego conflicts about status bulk larger as precipitation factors in accidents than conflicts about sexuality, even though occasionally a conflict about sex may provide the trigger reaction for the pattern of ill-considered aggressive or run-away behavior which eventuates in an accident.

The composite personality profile of the "accident-prone" individual has been described by Dunbar (17) as follows:
1. Far better than average health, with little tendency to colds, indigestion, stomach ulcers or other "vegetative" disturbances.
2. Impulsiveness of action under stress.
3. Failure to finish school.

4. Frequent change of jobs and many ups and downs in income.
5. Spontaneous and casual in social relations.
6. Apparently gets along well with members of the opposite sex, but irresponsible toward husband or wife or family.
7. Interest in machinery, sports and gambling.
8. No interest in philosophy beyond a firm belief in fate.
9. Makes up mind quickly.
10. Coffee, alcohol or cigarettes used to let off steam—not for sociability or to increase alertness or prolong working time.
11. Frequent conflicts with authorities. Attempt to deal with these by "being nice." Ignores existence of authority as long as possible.
12. History of broken homes—his parents' or his own.

The early expectation of Dunbar that patients with the accident habit could be diagnosed on the basis of their personality profile did not materialize. They learned that the seemingly "accident-prone" individual may have a series of mishaps in rapid succession, may go many years without one, or may never have another accident after the first. This paradoxical behavior of the "accident-prone" is attributed by Dunbar to their ability to develop psychological defenses against their emotional conflicts; they have an accident only when and if their defenses break down under strain.

The personality characteristics of the "accident-prone" persons, according to Dunbar, can be recognized at present only on the basis of their past record. This cautious statement is in sharp contrast to the more hopeful expressions contained in some of Dunbar's earlier studies: "Eighty to ninety per cent of all accidents are due to a personality factor which can be diagnosed before the habit develops, but which cannot be adequately dealt with by education or improvement of machinery."

The central focus of conflict of the "accident-prone" and the method employed in solving this conflict are described by Dunbar as follows: "The conflict between repressive authoritarian pressures and individual spontaneity is at least one factor which predisposes to accidents. Accident-prone individuals attempt to avoid or minimize conflicts with authority by focusing their values on immediate, concrete experiences, by avoiding any marked submission or domination in vocational and social roles and by striving for security and satisfactions outside of the authoritarian hierachy.

"When these usual defenses of the fracture patient fail and he can find no satisfactory escape from his hostility and guilt, his aggressiveness breaks out in an impulse to punish both himself and those responsible for his frustration. In the depressed individual, the suicidal attempt is usually a conscious experience. In the person with an accident syndrome, the process is brought about without conscious premeditation."

The "accident-prone" individuals tend to have accidents when "their strong aggressive hostility or resentment is aroused or the pressure from authority becomes too great. The various incidental and changing conditions play no part in accident-proneness, nor do reaction time, intelligence, physique or skill play any significant role."

In evaluating Dunbar's findings, it is well to bear in mind some of the limitations of her series. Like most accident studies, Dunbar's fractures are selective in some respects. The series was limited largely to one type of injury, to the ages of fifteen to fifty and to the white population of a metropolitan general hospital. The series is not particularly large for statistical purposes and was contrasted with several highly selective control groups, rather than with a general population. It may be worth noting that fractures constitute only about seven per cent of all injuries and that they are relatively more frequent among injured women than among injured men. Dunbar's conclusions that age and sex per se are relatively unimportant in the incidence of accidents are at variance with the findings of other investigators and are obviously due to the limitations of her series.

On the basis of preliminary studies the writer suspects that fracture patients, as a group, are more susceptible to multiple accidents than non-fracture patients or the population as a whole. Again, in the writer's experience, the personality profile attributed to the fracture group is not shared frequently by accident patients as a whole. The personality traits of Dunbar's fracture group seem to parallel the personality attributes of the writer's "maladjusted" group. The same characteristics were also encountered frequently in patients with other types of major injury, and less frequently in patients with repeated minor injuries.

It is often overlooked that Dunbar's conclusions are based primarily on extensive histories, although the findings "tended to be confirmed" later by a limited number of Rorshach tests and psychoanalytical studies. In summarizing her findings the author clearly points out that the personality profiles of the fracture patients were the least homogeneous among the five groups of illness studied.

Dunbar attributes "accident-proneness" to a conflict with authority which the individual is unable effectively either to avoid or to resolve. This theory of the dynamics of "accident-proneness" has been widely accepted, even though every conceivable type of psychological conflict has been implicated as possible factors in accident causation. It now seems evident that while specific psychological conflicts, especially conflicts with authority, play an important role in the causation of accidents, most psychologically determined accidents are due to non-specific or "free-floating" anxiety, produced by stresses and strains of everyday living.

Since the writer's studies indicate that the entire population is afflicted by accidents many times in the course of a lifetime, it follows that the personality types of accident patients as a whole are about as varied as the personality types of the total population.

The various specific psychological conflicts or traits which tend to increase susceptibility to accidents, and the personality characteristics and patterns of behavior which are frequently encountered in patients with repeated accidents, can admirably serve as diagnostic aids in the clinical diagnosis of the accident syndrome. The current restriction on the use of personality and behavioral data to attempts at diagnosing "accident-prone" individuals by means of specific personality profiles seems to place unnecessary limitations on highly useful diagnostic criteria.

Ackerman, Dunbar, Menninger, Rawson and others have described two types of benefit which the "accident-prone" patient may derive from his accident: (1) Primary gain—the accident serves the self-destructive tendency, the feelings of hatred and guilt and the need for punishment. Most people have the tendency to act out their feelings of hatred or guilt. The primary motive seems to be the expression of a self-destructive tendency due to guilt feelings or of a tendency to destroy others as an expression of hatred. Freud terms this acting out of the purposive destructive tendency 'the traumatophilic diathesis.' (2) Secondary gain—the accident helps the avoidance of disagreeable or dangerous situations, evasion of responsibility, monetary benefits, attention and sympathy. Secondary gain or motive closely is tied up with the personality of those who exhibit the primary motive in many instances.

In eighty to ninety per cent of the fracture patients studied by Dunbar some specific worry was reported preceding the accident. In many instances, the patient was doing something he was not sure was right, such as disobeying a parent, attempting independent behavior or avoiding authority. Frequently the patient expressed a feeling of guilt for behaving in this manner and said he deserved the accident: "It was really my fault because mother had said supper was ready and I was not to go out." The personality pattern of the person with an accident habit, says Dunbar, resembles that of the juvenile delinquent and adult criminal; however, one breaks laws and the other breaks bones.

In the writer's experience, the number of patients who give a history of anxiety or worry preceding an accident and who accept the injury as a deserved punishment is relatively small. This type of history is given more frequently by patients with a history of frequent accidents and is most common in patients with fractures and other serious injuries. This discrepancy in findings is probably more apparent than real and depends, perhaps, on differences in behavior following major and minor accidents. Patients with major accidents frequently express feelings of anxiety, guilt and deserved punishment soon after injury and retract or deny those feelings a day or so later. This strange behavior is perhaps due to the purifying effect of the major accident, on weakening of inhibitions and on putting the patient in a mood for confessing the otherwise suppressed feeling of guilt, anxiety, etc. The injury may represent coin paid to the super ego which buys permission to express impulses and conflicts previously repressed. By the same token, the minor accident probably lacks the necessary emotional ingredients to stimulate a confession and reveal the patient's subconscious thought processes.

The tendency of the severely injured person to confess fits in with the findings of Chamber and Reiser (13) in studies of acute cardiac patients in failure at the Cincinnati General Hospital. These patients were observed to confess a great deal of psychically meaningful material and two or three days later, when they were digitalized and compensated and presumably became completely "defended" again, denied the problems which previously they had brought forward.

There are patients who appear disappointed when informed that they have sustained only a minor injury, and there are those who will go to considerable lengths to deny the extent or severity of their injury. There are also patients who are unusually cheerful following an accident and whose behavior is quite out of keeping with the realities of the situation. This type of behavior is encountered in children as well as in adults, and in non-occupational as well as in occupational accidents.

The patients who appear disappointed by the fact that they did not have as severe an injury as they had thought, may actually have a tremendous need to bring out repressed material; but now that the injury was not great enough, they are unable to capitalize on the opportunity to let the repressed come forward. This denial mechanism is undoubtedly the same which people use in other circumstances when confronted with illness or problems and which some people use as a general stance; this mechanism is related, of course, to the magical period of childhood when things could be changed at will by now insisting on one thing and then another. The cheerfulness that was observed in this group of patients may in part represent the energy which was previously used to repress knowledge and which now has become available for euphoric purposes. The euphoria actually also may represent the sense of relief that the injury was not as complete and not as destructive or castrating as might have been unconsciously fancied.

Rawson (50) concludes that (1) a small number of people have multiple accidents whereas the majority have one accident or none; (2) the same groups with a high rate during one three-year period also had a high rate during the second period; (3) "accident-prone" individuals are "accident-prone" in any occupation; (4) a small group of people have a tendency to have multiple accidents and have the majority of all accidents; (5) accidents tend to predispose to more accidents, shortening the time between accidents, and (6) "accident-proneness" is a definite entity, concerns the individual exclusively and is not to any extent dependent upon the circumstances of environment at the time of the accident.

Rawson agrees that "accident-proneness" can be predicted at present only on the basis of past record. It has been shown, says this author, that "accident-prone" persons have certain definite characteristics of personality which if further studied may be of valuable aid to prediction. For the present, accidents due to "accident-proneness" may be prevented only by elimination of the "accident-prone."

About twenty-five per cent of workers are "accident-prone" states Forster (24). These have the most errors, poorest attendance records and react more slowly to supervision; they are inattentive, hurried, worried and subject to mental tensions. These characteristics are in turn dependent on deep-lying mental attitudes due to fear, depression, constant grudges, resentment toward bosses, domestic troubles, chronic alcoholism or subnormal mentality. They are sometimes exhilarated, unduly emotional or have an inferiority complex or an "it-cannot-happen-to-me" complex. All these, as well as mental fatigue, expose these workers to undue hazards.

Fetterman (22,23) agrees with Menninger that many "accident-prone" individuals subconsciously wish for some accident which can be explained on the basis of an attempt at partial suicide. Many such case histories have been given by Menninger. A four-way classification of causative factors of accidents has been suggested by Fetterman:

Type I —**Injury Neurosis:** The significant factor here is an actual change in the nervous system.
Type II —**Industrial Neurosis:** The most important element in this group is the individual's dissatisfaction at work and the escape which the injury offers.
Type III—**Indemnity Neurosis:** Motivated by a combat compensation.
Type IV—**Inherent Neurosis:** In which the pretraumatic personality was definitely nervous and the accident has

offered an opportunity to "project" the blame upon some other source.

In the historical sense, Type I covers "traumatic neurosis." The injury has resulted in physical distress, insomnia, weakness, irritability and disturbances of the psychic make-up. The second type is the most serious faced by Industrial Commissions. These individuals develop neurotic symptoms which have been responsible for disabilities extending into decades. While in many such patients the personality alone has been largely responsible, it is Fetterman's opinion that the work setting is the most significant cause of the chronic illness.

In a study of the neuropsychiatric aspects of industrial accidents, Fetterman states: "Disorders of the brain, disturbances of consciousness, disease of the spinal cord lead to unsteadiness, inattention, lapses, which result in accidents." Commonly, however, man-made accidents are the result of emotional and mental problems. The malingerer, the psychopath, the depressed patient is apt to have accidents which serve in an unconscious as well as in an objective way to provide (1) a solution for inner conflicts; (2) an escape for the individual; (3) revenge against authority, and (4) a means of self-punishment.

Wong and Hobbs (65) made a study to determine if the personality characteristics as noted by Dunbar in a hospital group were to be found in a high-accident group in industry. The study extended over two four-week periods. No attempt was made to identify the high-accident group on the basis of the interview and personal history alone. Seven personality traits, described by Dunbar as being characteristic of patients with multiple accidents, were studied in seventeen members of Group A with a high accident record as compared to a similar group having a low accident record during this period. Age was held constant, case histories and one-hour interviews were carried out for each man. They reported that the high and low-accident individuals differed markedly as a group in their personality traits and social adjustments. The high-accident worker came most frequently from a broken home and showed evidence of conflict with authority in both childhood and adulthood as revealed by truancy at school, contact with the Juvenile Court, a history of irregular work and of being fired, a record of marital discord and contact with social agencies. The low-accident worker, on the other hand, rarely showed difficulties of this nature in his life history. The authors agree with Dunbar that the aggressiveness which led to difficulties in their personal life is the same factor that produces a high accident record at work.

Adler (4) reported a study of one hundred and thirty American workers with repeated accidents. Certain recurring features were found, on the basis of which the cases were divided into eight groups as follows: revengeful attitude, "unlucky," longing to be pampered, overambitious, overfearful, alcoholic, feeble-minded and organic diseases. Adler remarks that while the average person avoids the possibility of accident, the "accident-prone" worker does not prevent accidents by this active, although frequently unconscious process.

In some of these accident-prone workers, states Adler, "the tendency to accidents disappeared after a fundamental change had been made in their lives. On the other hand, in many of the 'accident-prone' workers, injuries continued to occur even after they had been put to work where accidents were related to their personality rather than to the type of work. The majority of the one hundred and thirty workers examined were not suitable subjects for psychotherapy because of their bitter and hopeless attitude which would make any deep exploration an unpromising enterprise. It would be much easier to prevent their wrong development by adequate measures taken during childhood and adolescence."

Kunkle (38), who studied the psychological background of "pilot error" in aircraft accidents, agrees with most other observers that accidents are committed by a relatively small percentage of pilots. He concluded that psychiatric-psychological evaluation correlated significantly with susceptibility to "pilot-error" aircraft accidents. Present selection technics do not, however, predict "accident-proneness" in potential pilots. Two hundred AAF pilots (one hundred with histories of "pilot-error" accidents and one hundred control pilots) were examined with intensive, confidential interviews in an effort to uncover significant psychological correlates of flying accidents. It was discovered that (1) a past history of multiple fractures, dislocations and miscellaneous injuries; (2) the number of scars resulting from past accidents, and (3) ratings of "accident-proneness" by three independent judges correlate significantly with susceptibility to "pilot-errors" aircraft accidents. Falls down stairs, finger-caught-in-door accidents, auto accidents, and breaking of watch crystals are in general of negligible predictive value.

Horn (34) studied ten thousand aircraft pilots with two or more accidents in the air. He found that a pilot is much more likely to have another accident within thirty days of his first one—but the probability that a pilot will have another accident decreases markedly as time passes. The same phenomenon holds for later accidents, except that the later accidents occur even closer together than do the first two. The author does not feel that these findings can be explained entirely by hypotheses about poor pilot material or "accident-proneness," but possibly by the disruptive effect of an accident on the pilot's efficiency. As time goes on, the pilot regains his confidence and poise in the air and so is less likely to have an accident. Serious consideration should, therefore, be given to the readjustment of a pilot immediately following an accident. The accident habit is thus apparently a condition which is subject to ebb and flow and is governed by adaptability or adjustment to stressful situations.

Bond (12), in his book, *The Love and Fear of Flying,* points to war-time experiences which indicate that successful combat pilots were not necessarily the best adjusted individuals. A specific kind of maladjustment or character problem might actually enhance the pilot's effectiveness and render him less susceptible to injury and death.

Kemp (36), in a study of the human hazards in industrial employment, states that the emotional stresses involved in a job may be far more important than the physical stresses. Among the emotional disorders encountered are "accident-proneness," neurosis, traumatic neurosis, anxiety neurosis, conversion neurosis, compensation neurosis and conversion hysteria. The author makes an interesting observation in his discussion of compensation neurosis. Personal insult creates a center of turmoil in one's mind which is relieved or discharged, like a high potential of electricity or a head of steam, only by taking suitable retaliation or receiving an apology. Accidental injury (insult to soma) is similar in character to personal insult and the center of turmoil is discharged by compensation. Kemp's listing of various psychiatric problems in industrial employment leaves out the group which probably contributes the greatest number of accidents—the group of character neurosis or character disorders.

Sutter (69) calls accidents the "cancer of industry." He notes the fact that accidents cause the loss of thirty per cent more working years than cancer, and that the over-all industrial accident rate of two million per year has not been effectively reduced in years. He presents evidence to show that eighty per cent of the accidents arise from human failure and that ten per cent of the workmen contribute seventy-five per cent of the accidents. Sutter classifies the "accident-prone" into three groups: (1) those who have mental and physical defects; (2) those possessing insufficient skill or knowledge, and (3) those who have the so-called "improper attitudes." He believes that the third group, constituting the great majority of the "accident-prone" can be discovered by diligence and given more time, attention, training and supervision to reduce their "accident-proneness."

Giberson (28) states that nearly ninety per cent of industrial accidents are caused by emotional factors, of which fifty per cent may be avoided through preventive medicine. Near accidents and narrow escapes are not generally reported, yet emotional shock and damage are great, and unless treated bring loss of time, skill and efficiency, and may leave a predisposition to accidents and may even develop into an anxiety neurosis.

Csillag and Hedri (14) studied a group of patients with recurrent accidents due to personality factors and found that fifty-four per cent of the patients had lost one of their parents in childhood through death or separation. Almost one-third of the patients' deceased fathers had been the victim of violent death, compared to 0.06% of the average population. Forty per cent worked in fields unsuitable for their emotional constitution. Seventy per cent of the patients could not give free expression to their aggressive drives in any other way except through an accident, even though some tried to do so by choice of vocation, through indulging in sports and by other means. These authors conclude that the motive of accidents is aggression turned against one's self, that the causes of accidents are of manifold determination and that breaks in the relation of child and parent are of decisive effect. They recommend preventive personality examinations and emotional treatment after accidents.

A description of the personality of the "accident-prone" individual by Alexander (6) may be summarized as follows: The "accident-prone" person is decisive or even impulsive and is apt to act upon the spur of the moment. He likes excitement and adventure and does not like to plan and prepare for the future. This impetuousness may have various reasons, but apparently rebellion against restrictions by authority and all forms of external coercion is its most common origin. At the same time, he has a strict conscience which makes him feel guilty for this rebellion. In the unconsciously provoked accident, the "accident-prone" expresses his resentment and revenge, at the same time atoning for his rebellion by his injury. A large number of persons with the accident habit has had a strict upbringing and has derived from this an unusual amount of resentment against persons in authority. The "accident-prone" person is essentially a rebel. He cannot even tolerate self-discipline and rebels not only against external authorities, but against the rule of his own reason and self-control toward his parents. The combination of these two, resentment and guilt, says Alexander, is the most common factor in accidents.

3. PSYCHODYNAMICS OF ACCIDENTS IN CHILDREN

Klein (37) believes that certain so-called accidents in children, especially certain forms of self-injury, are determined by obscure psychological factors. "A tendency to plaintiveness in children and a habit of falling down and knocking or hurting themselves are to be regarded as expressions of certain fears and feelings of guilt . . . . such recurrent minor accidents and sometimes more serious ones are substitutes for self-inflicted injuries of a graver kind, and may represent attempts at suicide with insufficient means."

Schmideberg (52) considers accidents to be one of the many subconscious substitutes for suicidal phantasies. Suicidal tendencies (as well as accidents), says this author, are less common in childhood than in adult life, partly because of the greater measure of success with which reality is denied in childhood.

Putnam and Stevens (49) in a study of the mental life of the child declare that hostile feelings in an older child are noticeable on the arrival of a new baby. "For many children the thought of the approaching arrival of a little brother or sister is so exciting that they threaten to throw the child into the water or else 'to put the baby under the bed,' the place where the child tucks away unpleasant things out of sight. A little lad forced into the background by his small sister, intentionally hurt himself by letting himself fall from a chair: but then, when caressed by his parents, he admits, while weeping—from pain or for joy, 'I did it on purpose.'"

Ackerman and Chidester (4) attribute the "accident-proneness" of children to indulgence in habitually reckless play as a result of such emotional factors as fear, unexpressed hatred and feelings of guilt. "Injury causes the child to receive attention and sympathy, but there are also indirect benefits, such as avoidance of disagreeable situations and evasion of responsibility. Hurting himself and thus relieving this sense of guilt is probably primary."

In a study of the incidence of first aid treatments in children, Fuller (27) found that referrals to first aid were not distributed evenly among the children, but showed from the early age of two how children vary, from those who monopolize the nurse's time to those who are never seen by her. Girls are more sharply divided into injury-prone and non-prone than are boys.

Fuller further reports that there is a poor correlation between injuries and intelligence. He suggests that those children who get hurt most often may have more problematic behavior. The injury-prone children tend to be injured more frequently themselves, but do not necessarily cause injuries to others. "There appears to be considerably more than age, intellect, sex or isolated personality traits operating to produce the injury-prone or non-injury-prone child. This complexity of the problem is in accord with the findings in the accident-prone adult."

Fabian and Bender (19) studied eighty-six children with severe head injuries on the Children's Psychiatric Service of Bellevue Hospital; they found that thirty-three of the children, or thirty-eight per cent, had been involved in two or more major accidents and could be described as suffering from an accident habit. The children studied were one to fifteen years of age, of whom ninety-two per cent were boys. The highest number of accidents occurred in the children five to six years of age.

These authors reported psychopathologic disorders in the parents of eighty-three per cent of the children who had the accident habit. In nearly half of these cases, one or both parents were alcoholic. In many instances the fathers were domineering, abusive and rejecting, the mothers submissive and overprotecting. The fathers were shiftless and economically incapable. Violent displays of temper were common as were marital disharmony, disruption of family life by hospitalization and jail sentences, as well as broken homes. The children were confused. Rejection, abuse and neglect intensified their aggressive drives.

Fabian and Bender found that a strong sadomasochistic behavior pattern accounted for the most characteristic profiles of their group. They compare accidents in young children to delayed temper tantrums and believe that accidents represent inverted aggressive gestures aimed at frustrating adults. Self-inflicted injuries due to depressive states were met occasionally. They attribute some accidents in childhood to sibling rivalry, the acting out of Oedipal conflicts, and to problems arising out of identification with the aggressor. It is common for children, when they feel that they are treated unfairly, to wish they were sick or dead so that their parents would feel sorry for them. With the large majority of children, these ideas are transient and are not acted upon. However, some children do act out their fantasies and then an "accident" may result.

When children are exposed to a sadistic father and a masochistic mother, the child reflects in his behavior the sado-masochistic conflict. His attitude toward his parents distorts his Oedipal strivings during the critical period of psychosexual development. Mounting anxiety and guilt interfere with his relationship to his parents and are carried over to the people with whom he comes in contact outside the home. He is unable to experience positive feelings without hostile overtones, so that all his relationships have a sadomasochistic quality. He welcomes pain to achieve his balance or to assuage his guilt, or even because, like the gambler or mountain-climber who courts danger, he has perversely eroticized anxiety itself. These children, say Fabian and Bender, are confused in their interpersonal relationships. Accustomed to an atmosphere in which power is the dominant note, their whole behavior, patterned on this model, is heavily tinctured with aggression. The abuse and rejection they suffer intensifies their aggressive drives. Since open expression of hostility is not tolerated and retaliation is impossible, the child's aggression is constantly backfiring. This sequence is commonly observed in the temper tantrum where the young child, unable to give vent to his hostility, often injures himself; he beats his head on the ground in a token display of his aims toward the frustrating adult. Self-injury used as an aggressive weapon is characteristic of the young child.

The psychodynamics of frequent accidents in children is summarized in a paper by Bakwin and Bakwin (8). The outstanding feature in the development of the "accident-prone" is a conflict with authority. This begins with a conflict involving the authority of the parents or stepparents, next at school, later with church and employer and finally in the marital relationship. Resistance to authority is particularly frequent in children who are brought up in a home where one or both parents are over-authoritative. Rejection is often associated with over-authority. The revolt against over-authority manifests itself during childhood by restless behavior, lying, stealing and truancy, but these tendencies disappear later on.

Some children, when criticized or scolded, or when they feel that they have been treated unjustly, obtain relief from pent-up aggression by striking inanimate objects, at times sustaining an injury in this way. Others, under similar circumstances, put themselves in dangerous situations. Jealous children sometimes inflict injuries on their younger siblings, especially when the younger sibling is rejected by the parents. A high percentage of accidents in children occur when they are doing things forbidden by their parents.

In those accidents which result from psychological conflicts, psychological needs may influence the accident in two ways: first, there may be what has been already referred to as an actual need for punishment, with all the implications thereof. Again, the accident may be an incidental product of a character defense mechanism in which the individual reacts to a life situation in accordance with his needs, and this reaction leads him into situations or circumstances which involve him in accidents.

In the aforementioned second instance, the accident does not fulfill any particular need as such, but is rather the outgrowth of a requirement for certain types of activity which secondarily involves the person in accidents. This type of individual technically called by some, the "phallicnarcissistic character," has a constant demand to reassure himself and to relieve his castration anxiety and to this end he engages in extremely hazardous types of occupations and acts. This type of person has no particular call to be injured and the greater incidence of accidents in this group is probably a reflection of their greater concern in exposure to hazards and not of a greater desire to be injured.

The high accident frequency of young adults in the early twenties may be related to this same purpose to court danger. It is around this age that the whole of the narcissistic and heterosexual problems come forth and young persons pass on to a more completely heterosexual form of existence and to a less narcissistic type of dynamic motivation.

It might help to clarify thinking if we were to consider such patients, whose accidents or injuries are in the nature of a compulsion to satisfy unconscious psychological needs, as suffering from a kind of neurosis. This syndrome should perhaps be designated as accident neurosis, or traumatophilic neurosis, to distinguish it from multiple accidents without neurosis and from neuroses without traumatophilia. Accident or traumatophilic neurosis need not be confused with "traumatic neurosis" which is, by definition, an entirely different, reactive clinical entity.

On the basis of his clinical experience and studies, this writer is inclined to believe that accidents due to specific or deep psychological problems are relatively infrequent. Most accidents of psychogenic etiology are probably due to non-specific emotional factors and are related to trials of everyday life. It should, perhaps, be emphasized that in most of the accidents in which psychological factors play either minor or major roles, it is not the accident or the injury per se that the individual is seeking. The accidents are merely an indirect outgrowth of circumstances or situations that the individual gets into because of psychological demands.

CHAPTER FOUR

CHARTS AND TABLES

Several of the chapters of this text make reference to the same tables and charts. On this account it has been deemed preferable not to locate tables and charts in the chapter of their chief use nor to repeat in others referring to them. Instead, all major arrangements in tabular form and charts have been segregated as shortly to follow. These statistical compilations are selective in that they fail to preempt the total lot prepared. Hope is that future publications as now planned may provide additional arrangements supplementing the already large number here introduced.

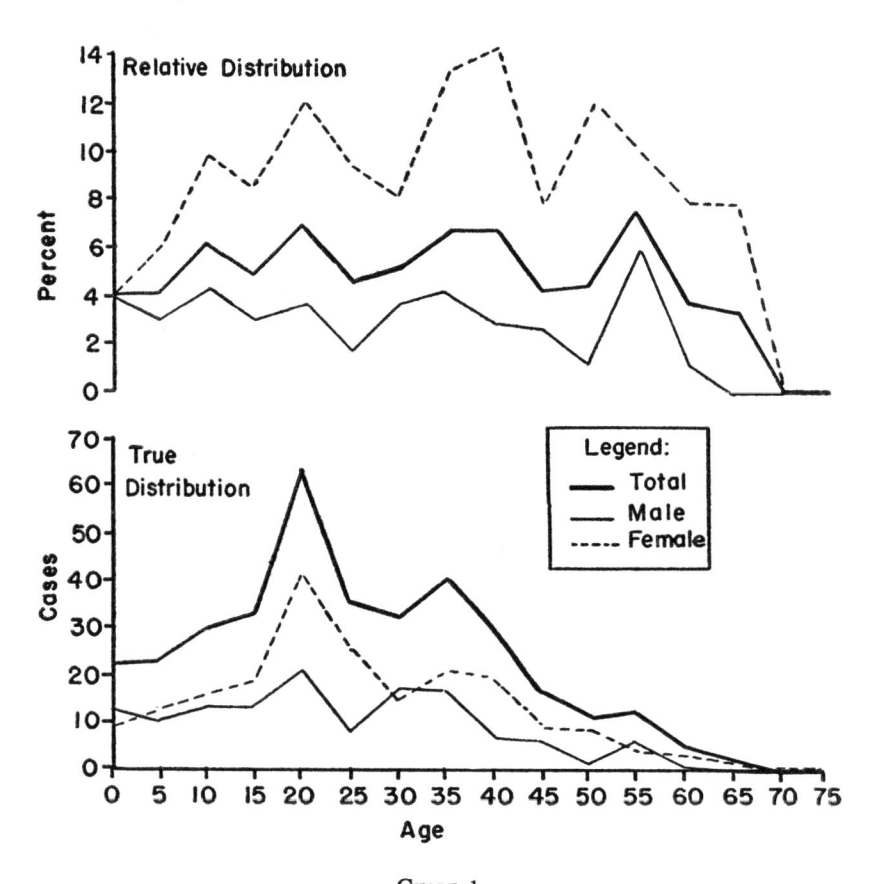

CHART 1

CASES FROM HANDLING HOUSEHOLD UTENSILS AND THEIR RELATIVE DISTRIBUTION
BY AGE AND SEX
NON-INDUSTRIAL 1930-1948

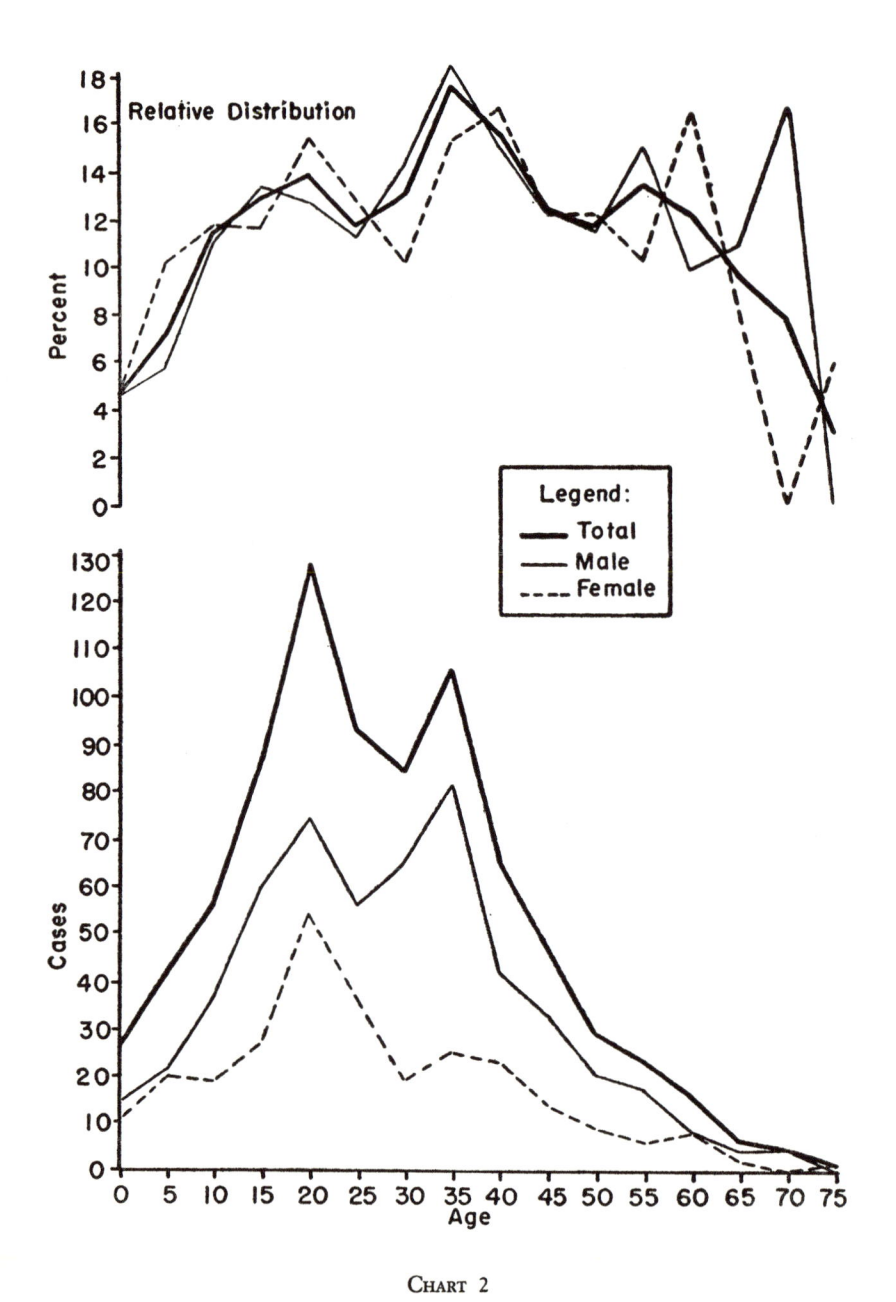

CHART 2

CASES FROM HANDLING OBJECTS, INCLUDING HOUSEHOLD UTENSILS, AND THEIR
RELATIVE DISTRIBUTION BY SEX AND AGE
NON-INDUSTRIAL 1930-1948

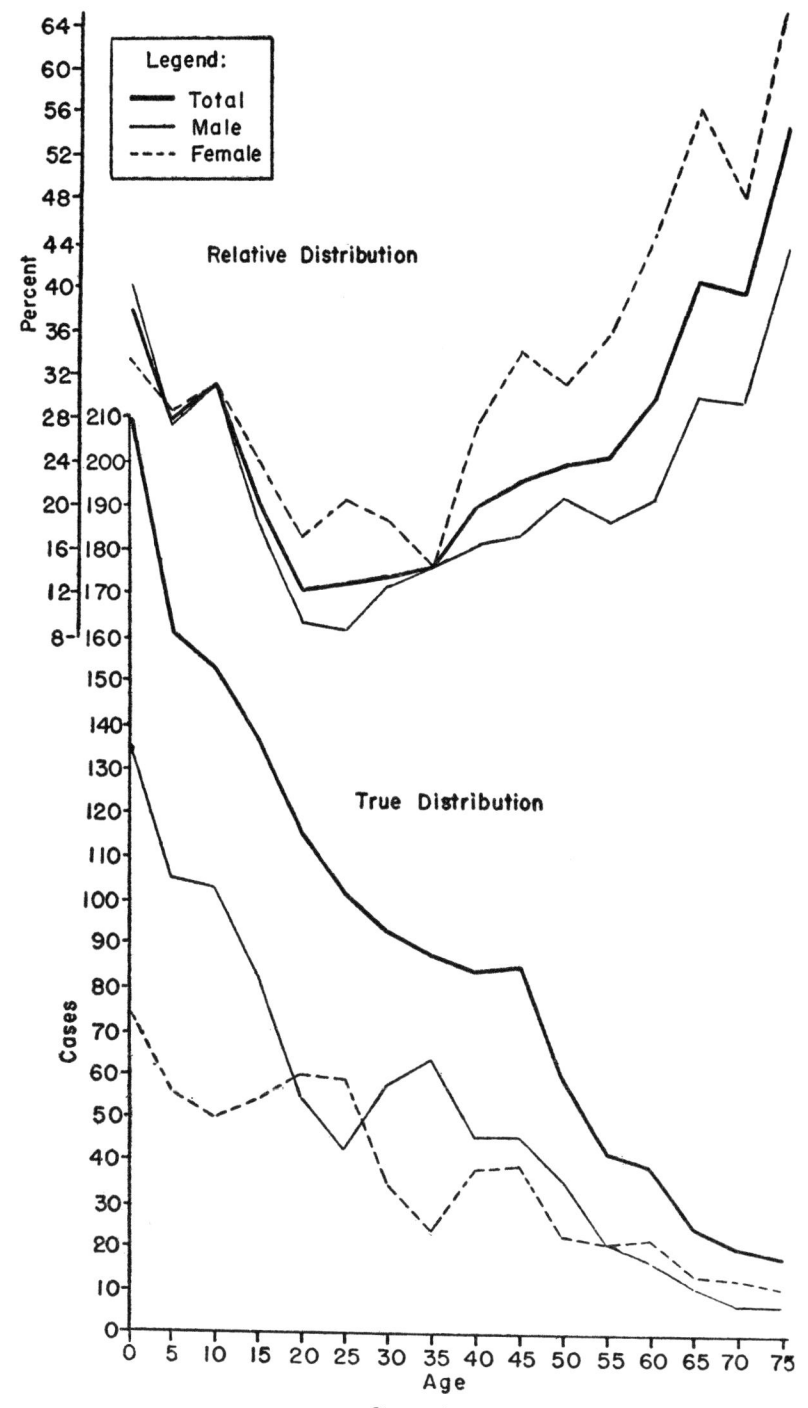

CHART 3
CASES FROM FALLS AND THEIR RELATIVE DISTRIBUTION BY AGE AND SEX
NON-INDUSTRIAL 1930-1948

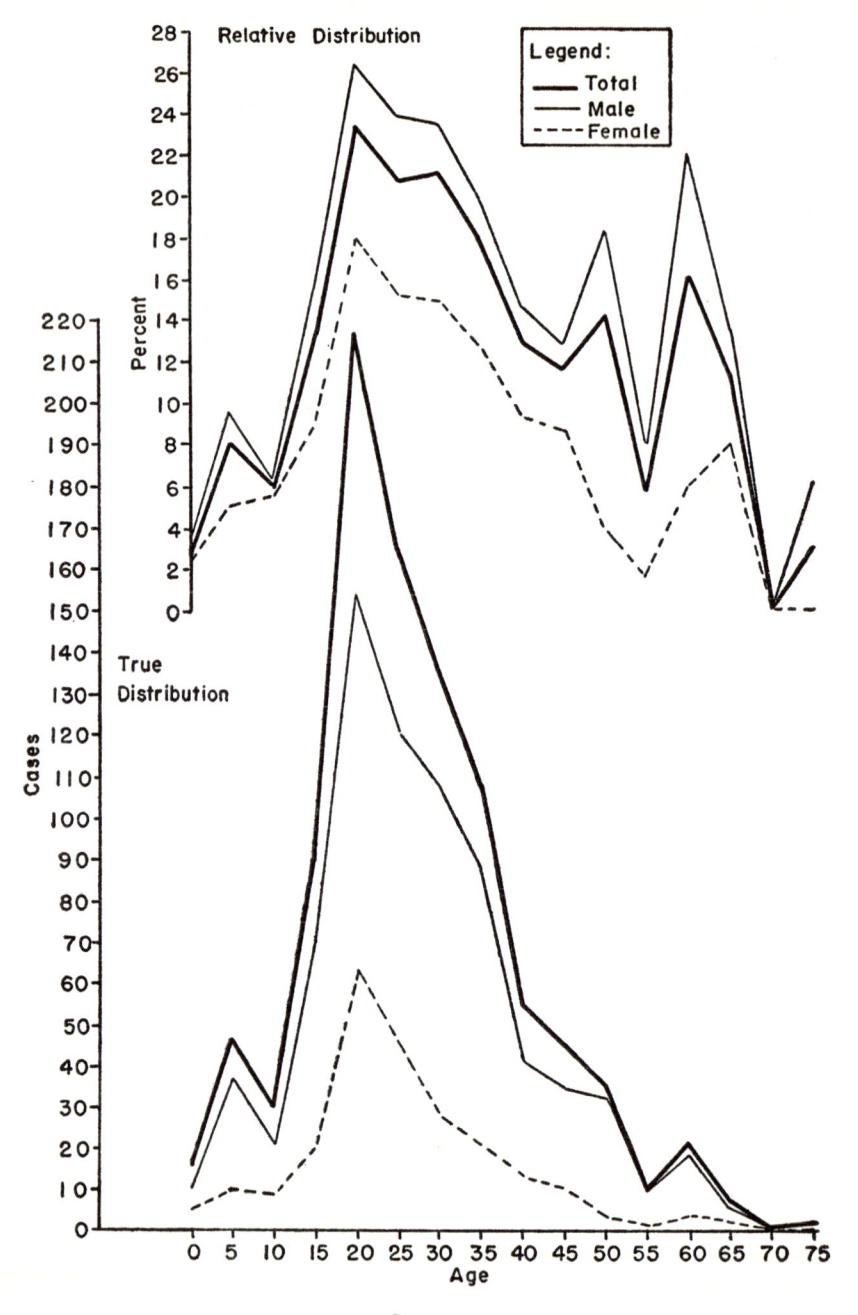

CHART 4

CASES FROM AGGRESSION (FIGHTS AND ATTACKS) AND THEIR RELATIVE DISTRIBUTION
BY SEX AND AGE
NON-INDUSTRIAL 1930-1948

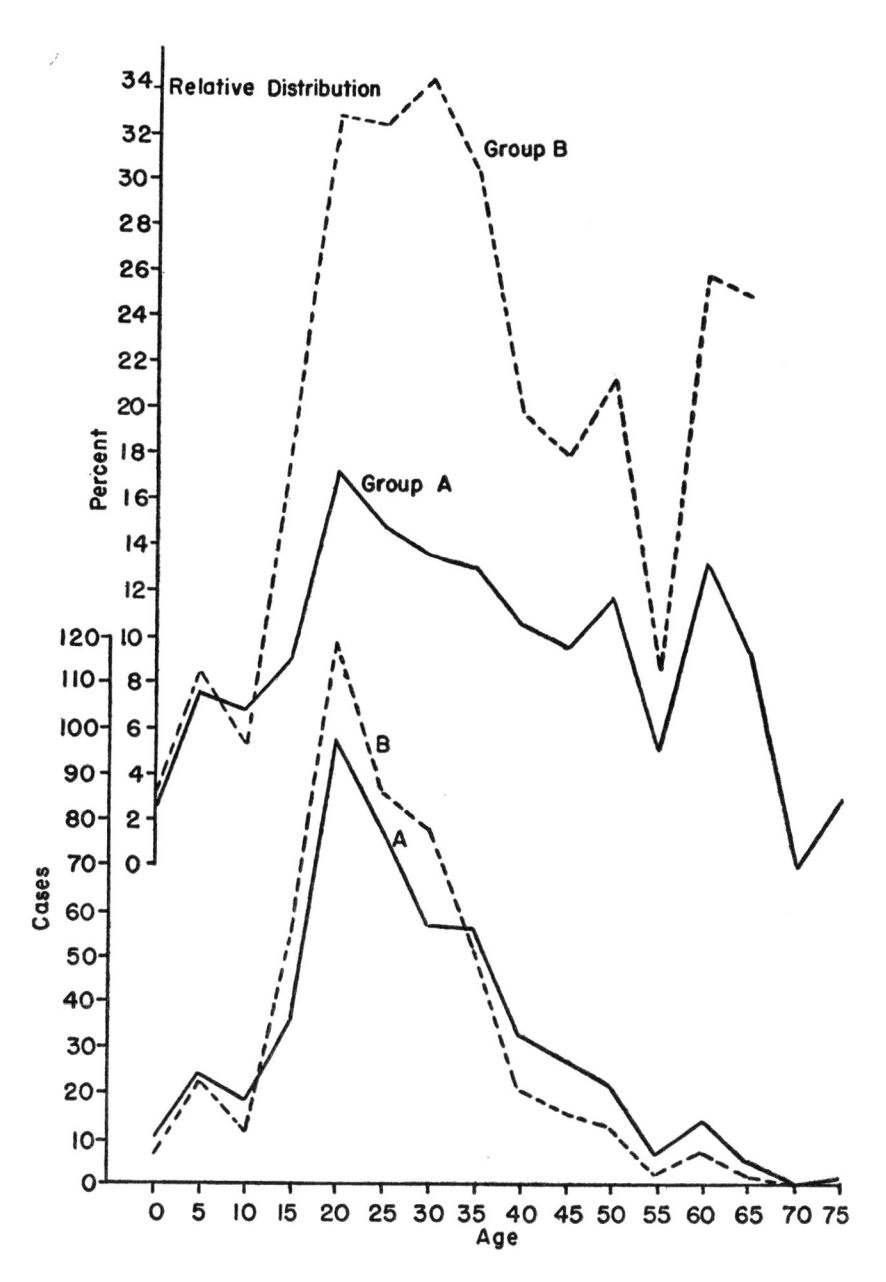

CHART 5

CASES FROM AGGRESSION (FIGHTS AND ATTACKS) AND THEIR RELATIVE DISTRIBUTION
BY AGE
NON-INDUSTRIAL GROUPS A AND B 1930-1948

Foreign Bodies

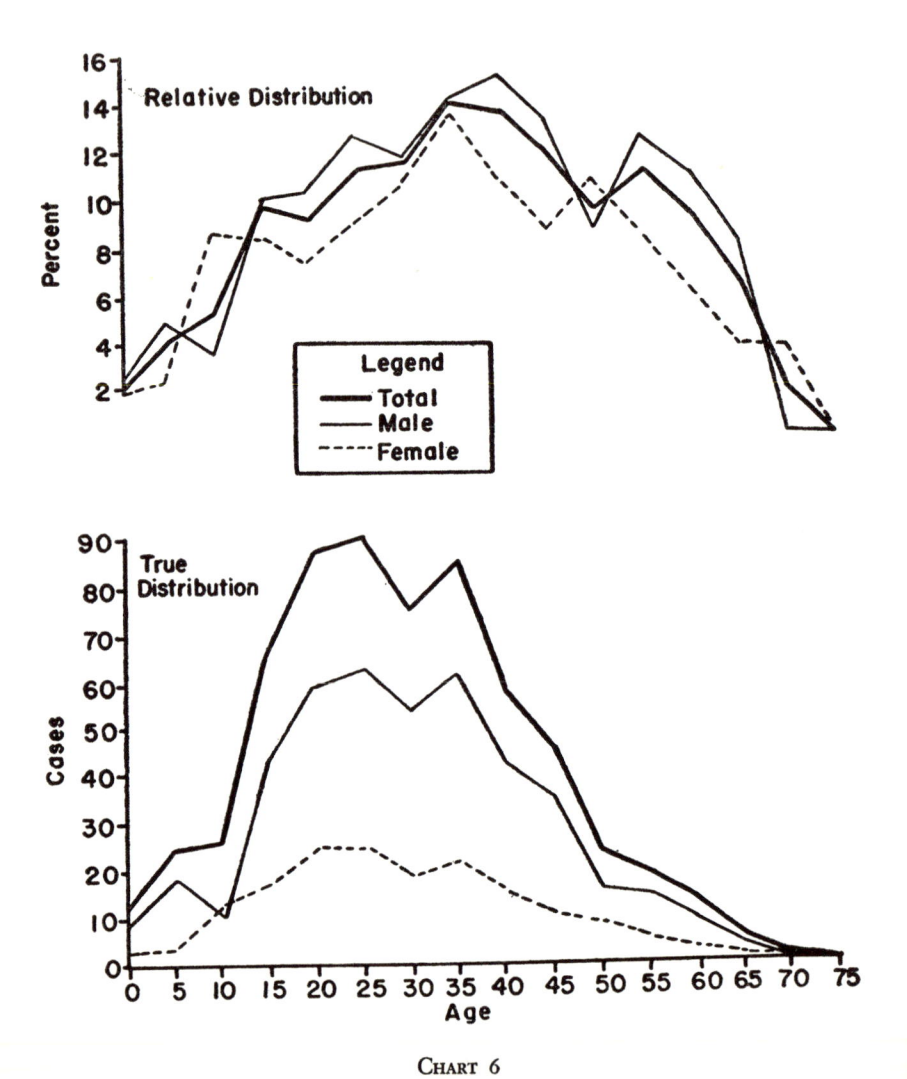

CHART 6

CASES FROM FOREIGN BODIES AND THEIR RELATIVE DISTRIBUTION BY SEX AND AGE
NON-INDUSTRIAL 1930-1948

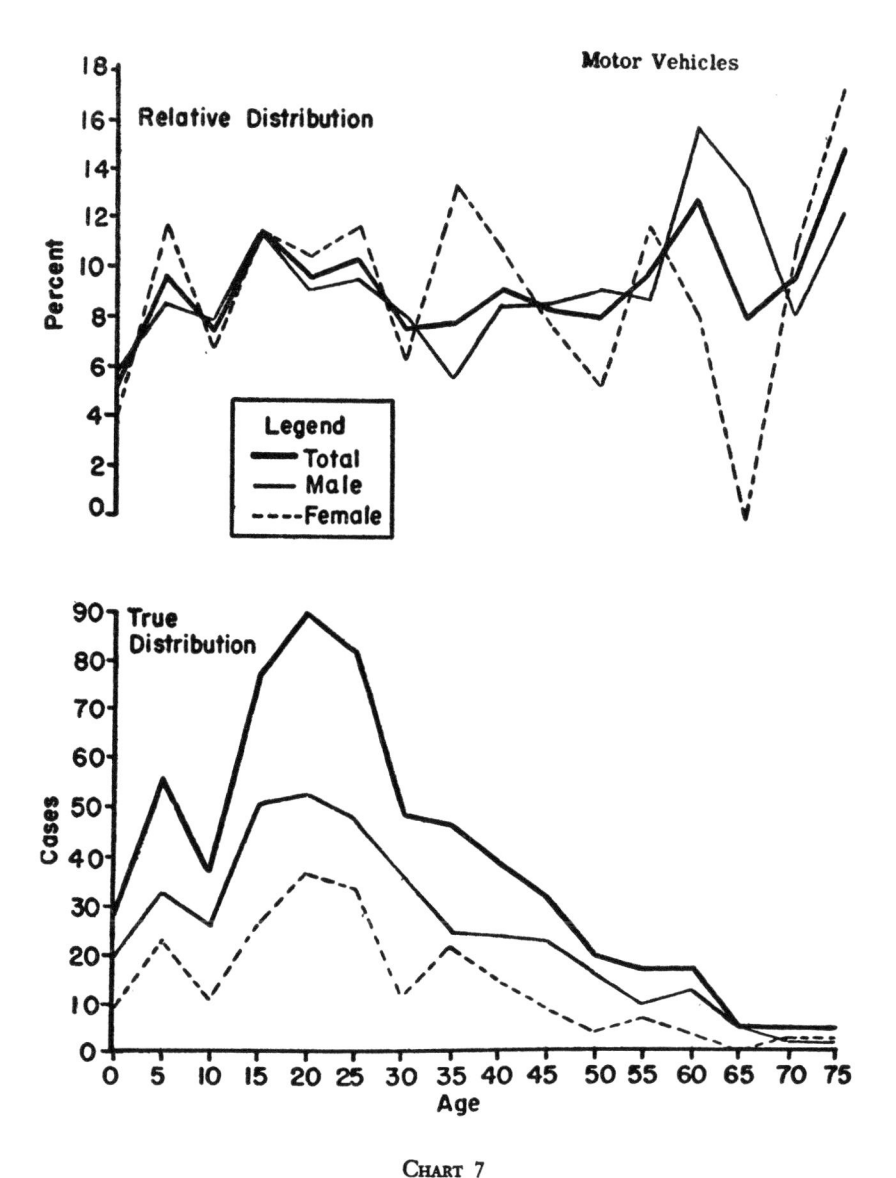

CHART 7

CASES FROM MOTOR VEHICLES AND THEIR RELATIVE DISTRIBUTION BY SEX AND AGE
NON-INDUSTRIAL 1930-1948

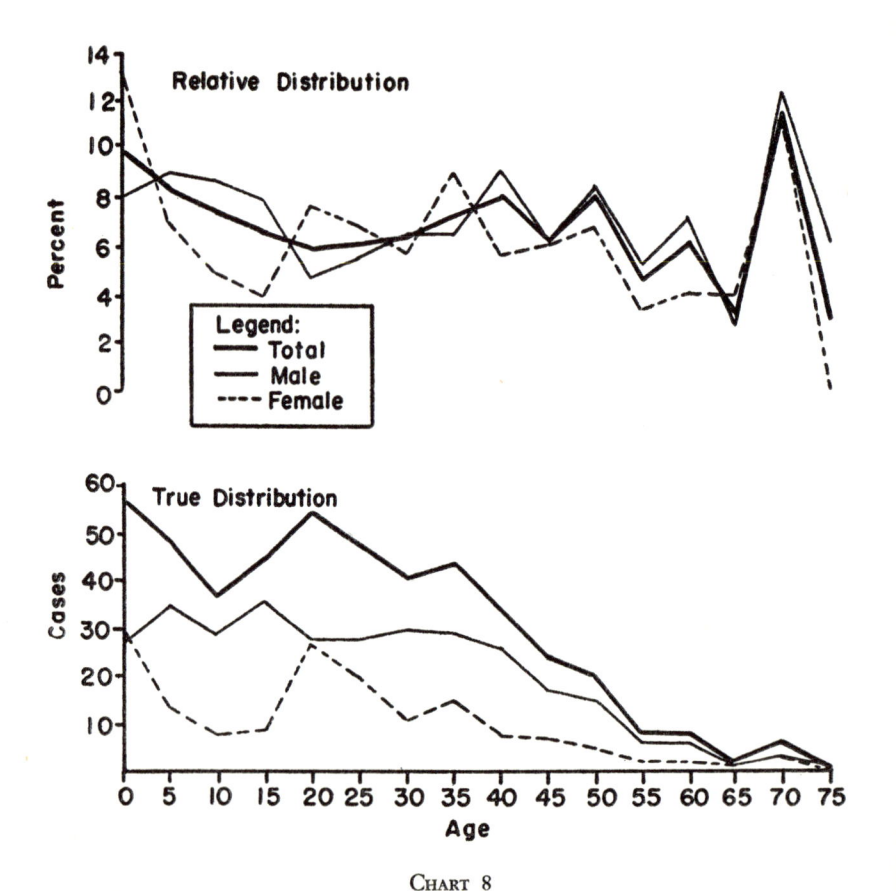

Bumping into Objects

CHART 8

CASES FROM STUMBLING AND THEIR RELATIVE DISTRIBUTION BY AGE AND SEX
NON-INDUSTRIAL 1930-1948

CHART 9

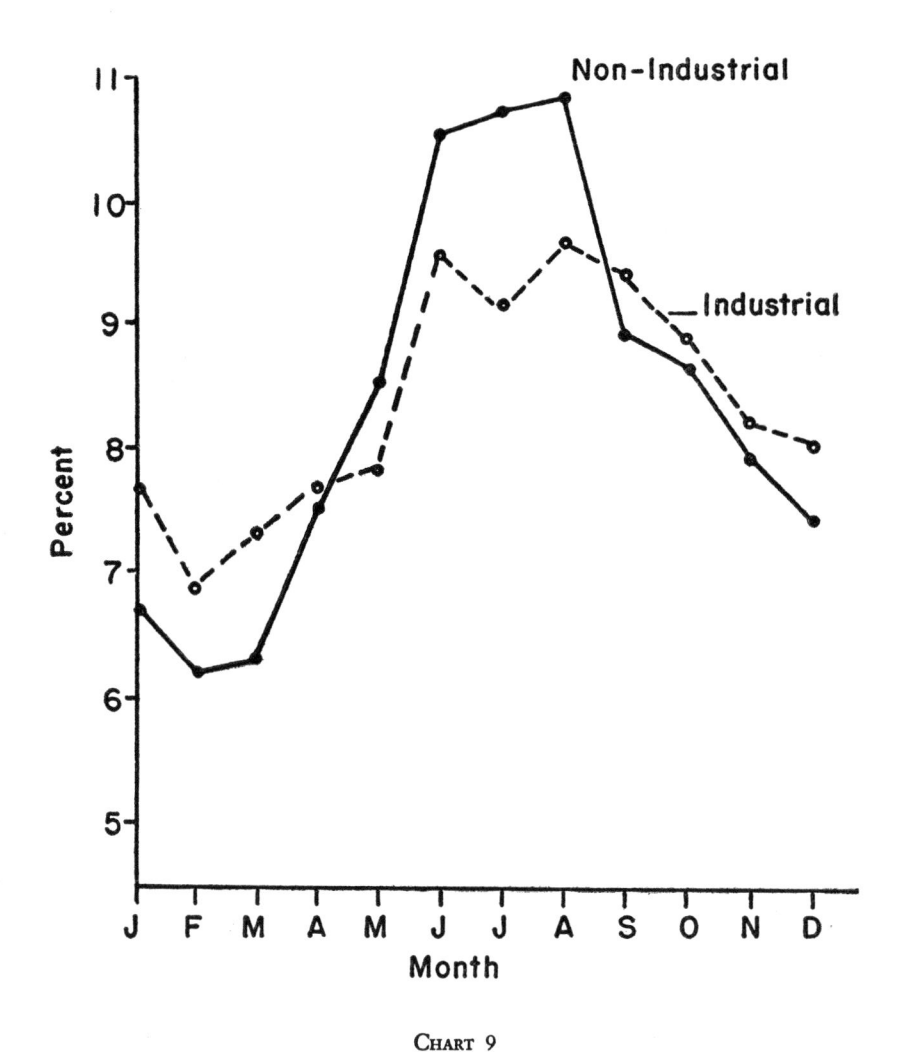

INDUSTRIAL ACCIDENTS (1942-44 and 1946-48) AND NON-INDUSTRIAL ACCIDENTS (1930-1948) BY MONTH OF OCCURRENCE — ALL AGES

CHART 10

Percentage of Non-Industrial Accidents by Months and Age 1930-1948

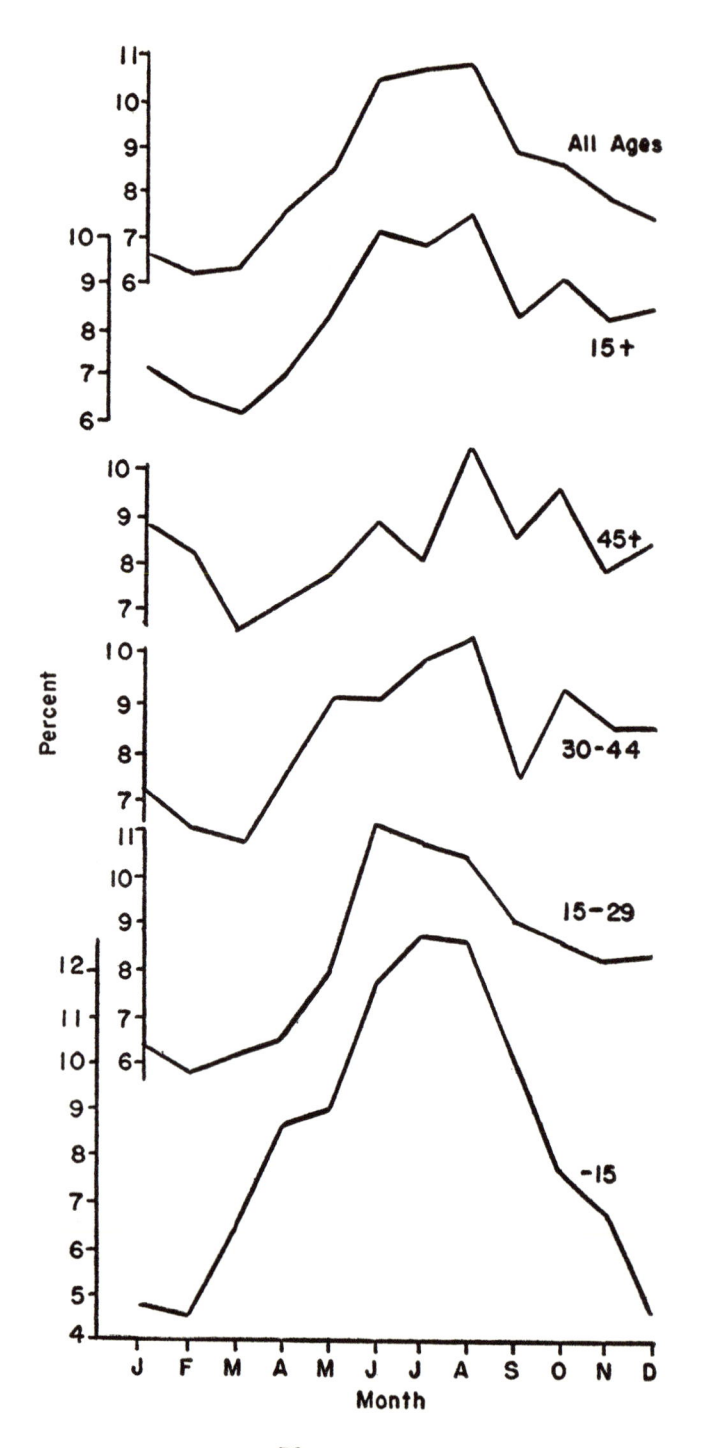

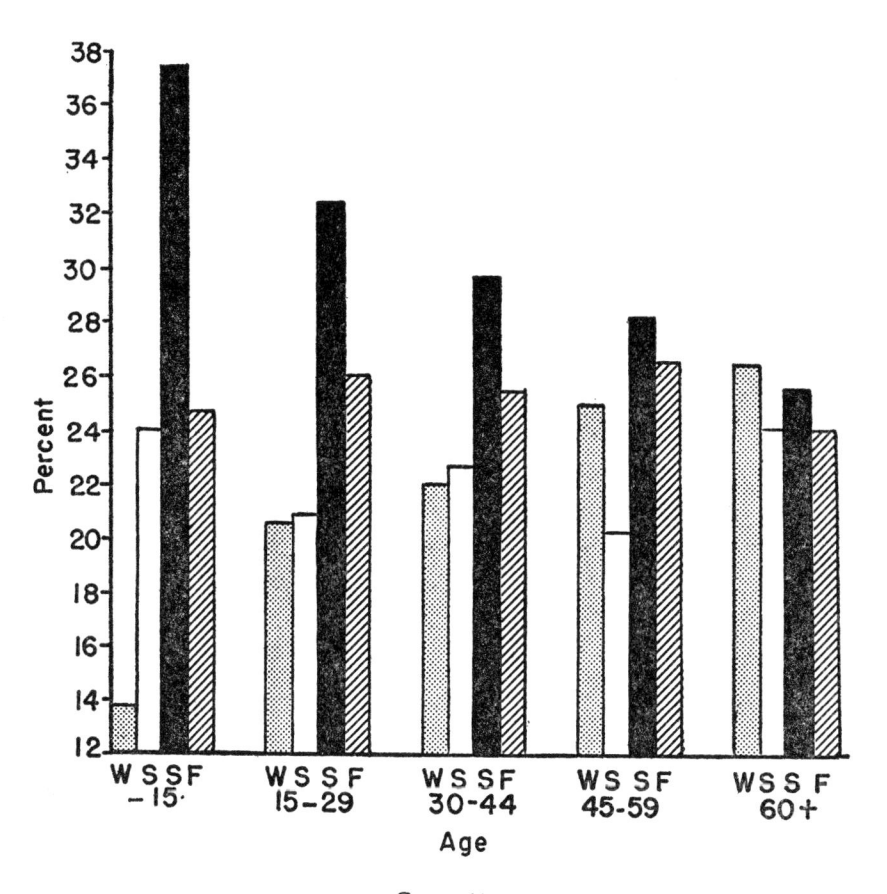

CHART 11

PERCENTAGE OF NON-INDUSTRIAL ACCIDENTS BY SEASON AND AGE 1940-1948

CHART 12

PERCENTAGE OF MALE NON-INDUSTRIAL ACCIDENTS BY AGE AND MONTH 1930-1948

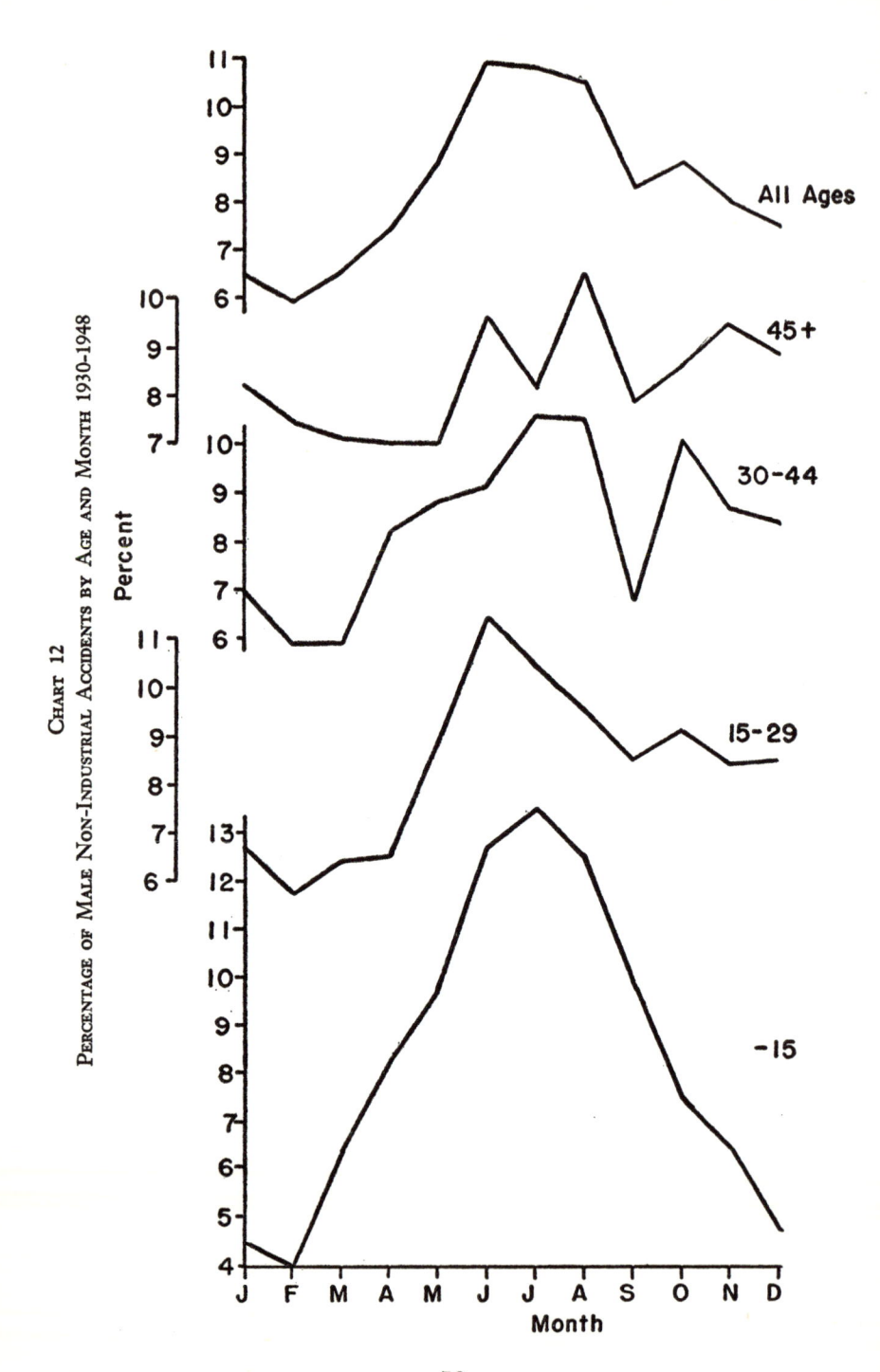

CHART 13

PERCENTAGE OF FEMALE NON-INDUSTRIAL ACCIDENTS BY AGE AND MONTH 1930-1948

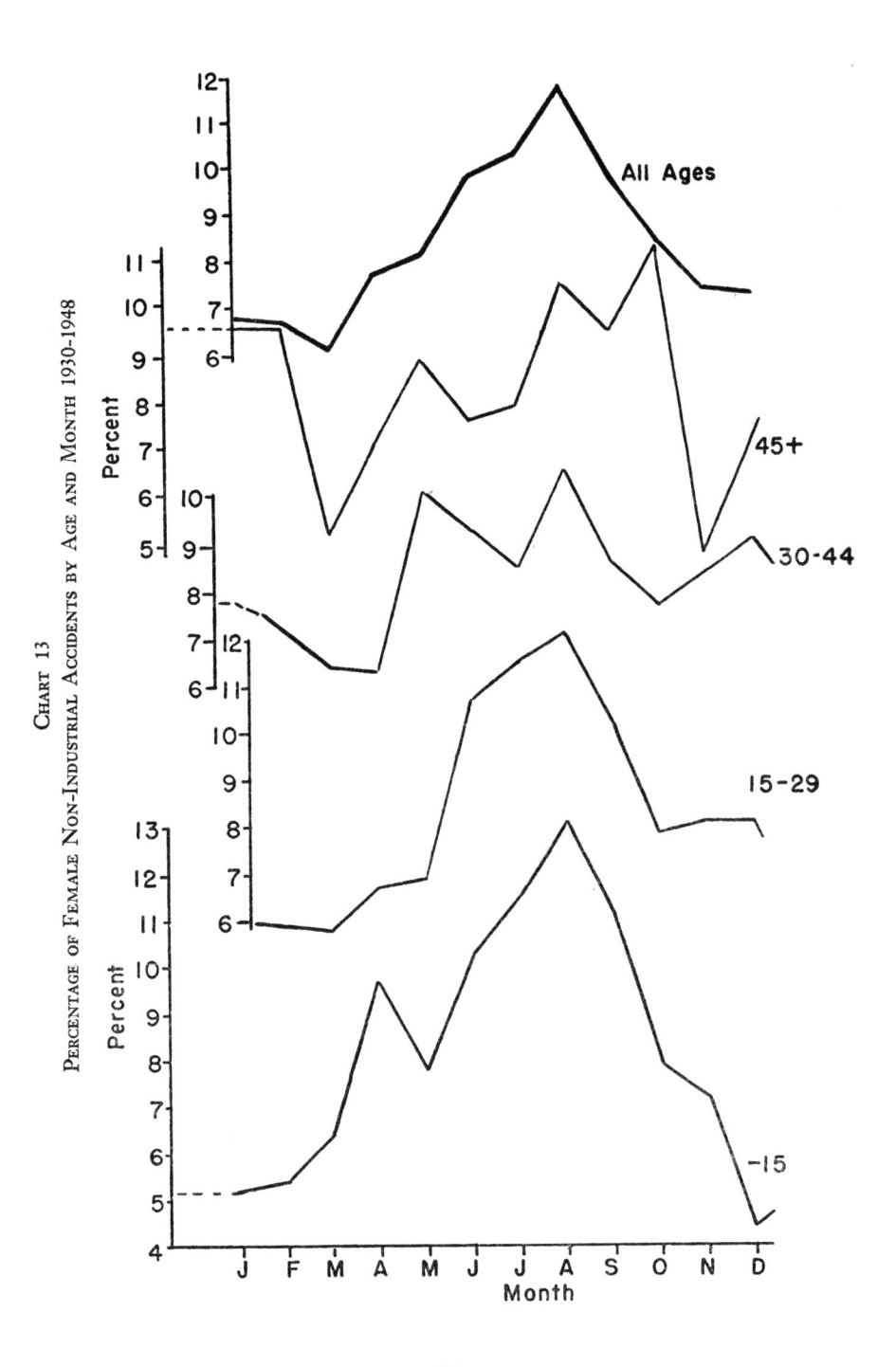

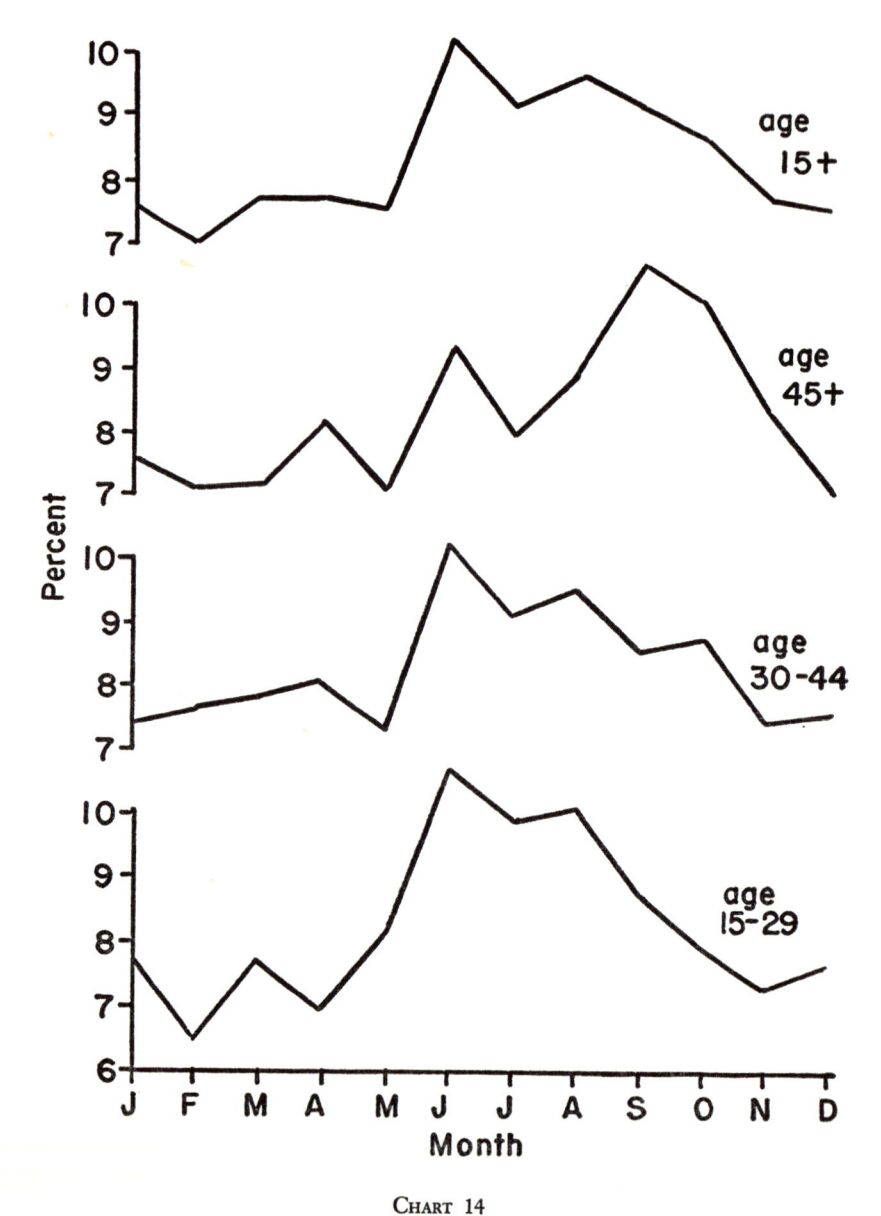

CHART 14

PERCENTAGE OF INDUSTRIAL ACCIDENTS BY MONTH AND AGE 1942-1944

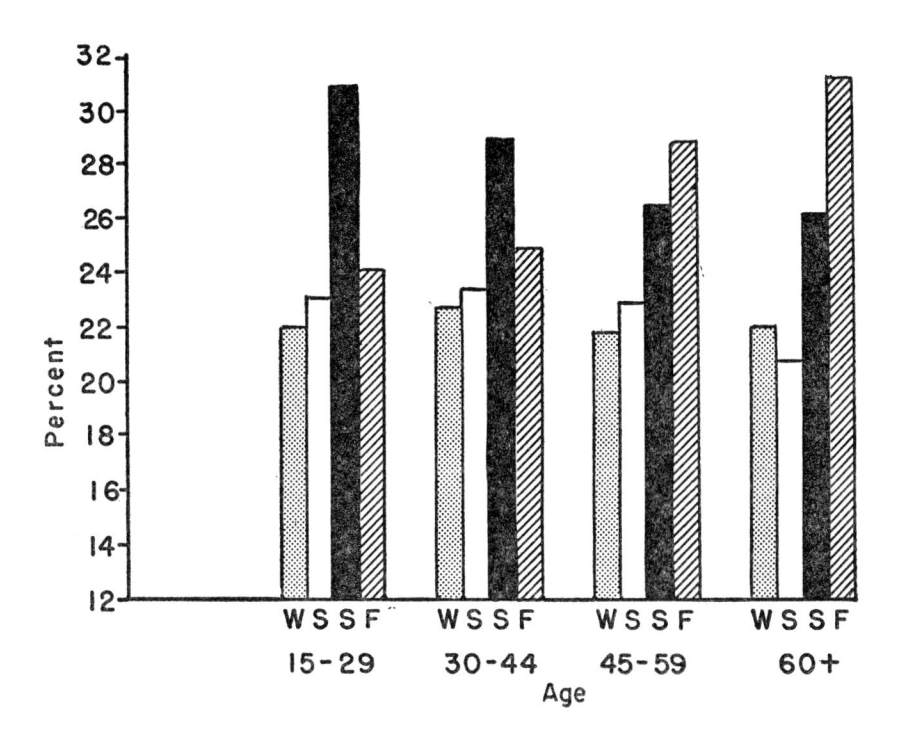

CHART 15

PERCENTAGE OF INDUSTRIAL ACCIDENTS BY SEASON AND AGE 1942-1944

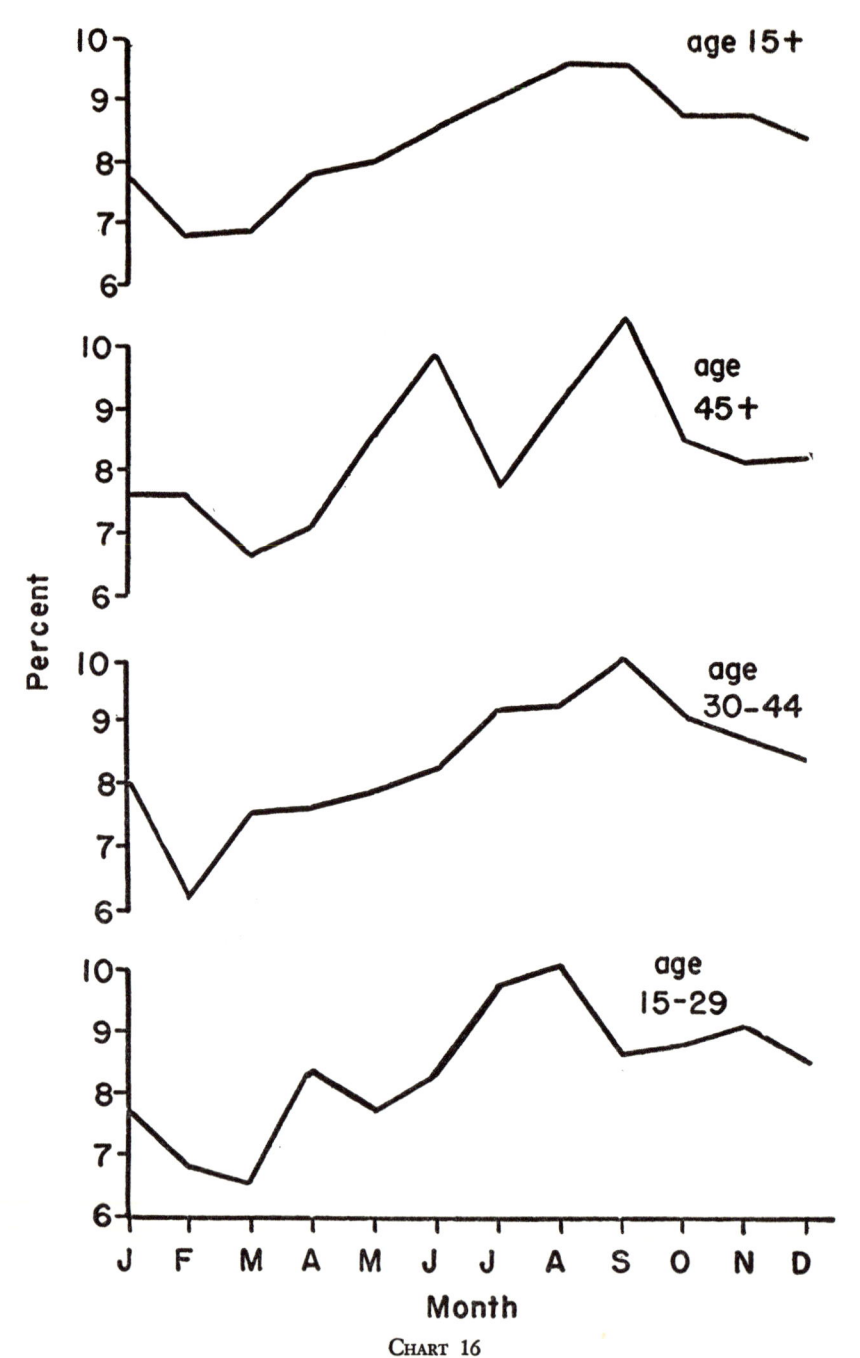

CHART 16
PERCENTAGE OF INDUSTRIAL ACCIDENTS BY MONTH AND AGE 1946-1948

CHART 17
PERCENTAGE OF MALE INDUSTRIAL ACCIDENTS BY MONTH AND AGE 1942-44
1946-48 SERIES COMBINED

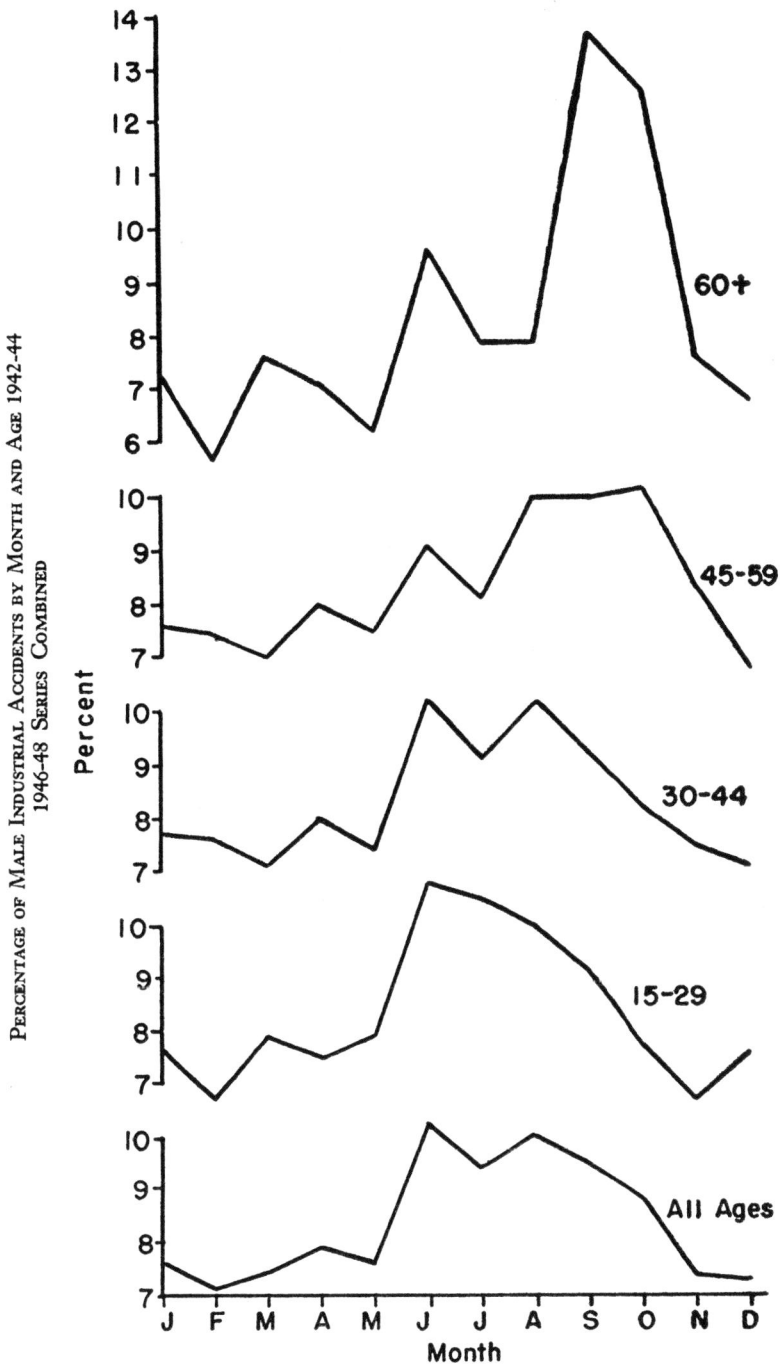

CHART 18
PERCENTAGE OF FEMALE INDUSTRIAL ACCIDENTS BY MONTH AND AGE 1930-1948

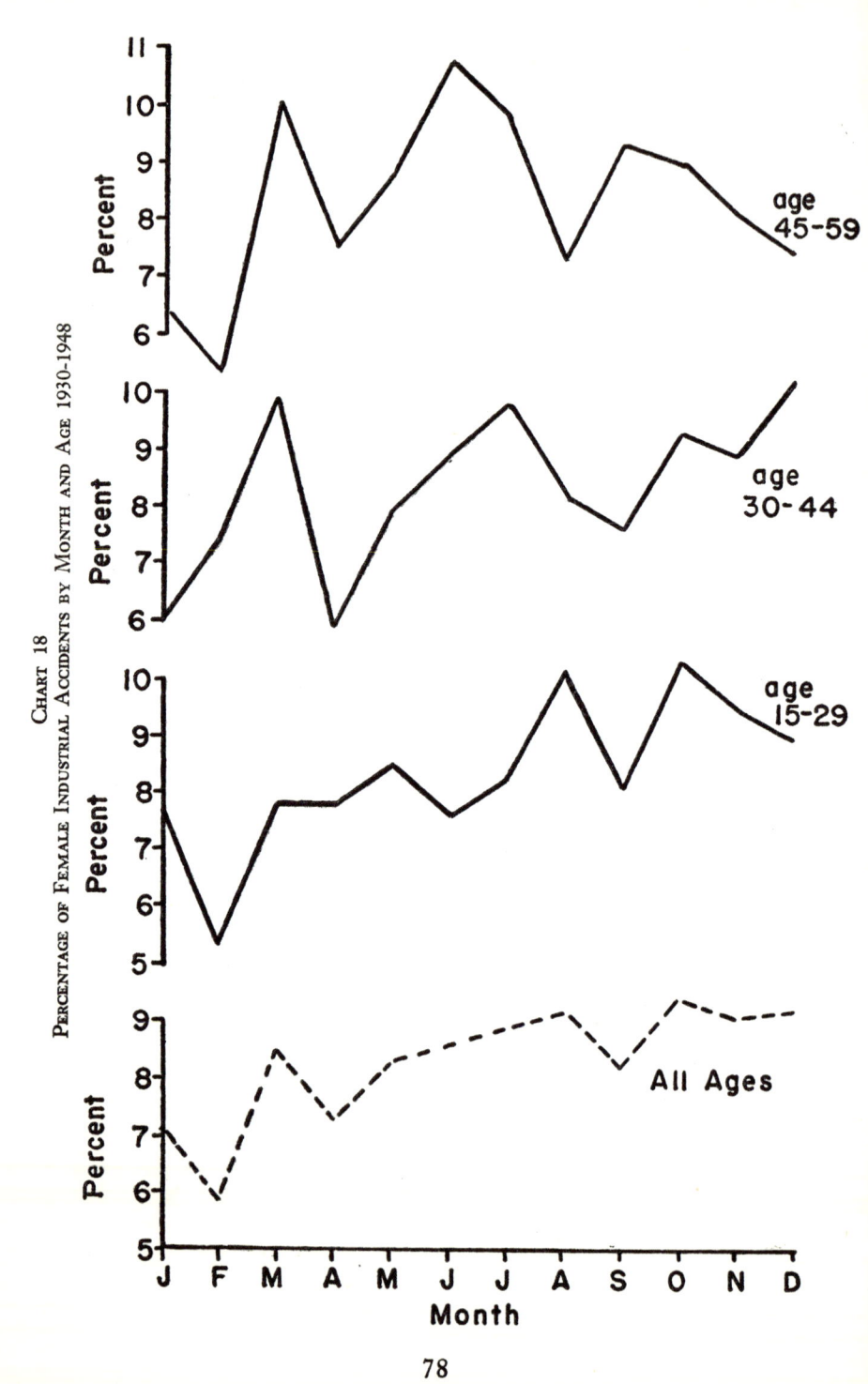

CHART 19

HOUR OF NON-INDUSTRIAL ACCIDENTS BY SEX 1930-1948

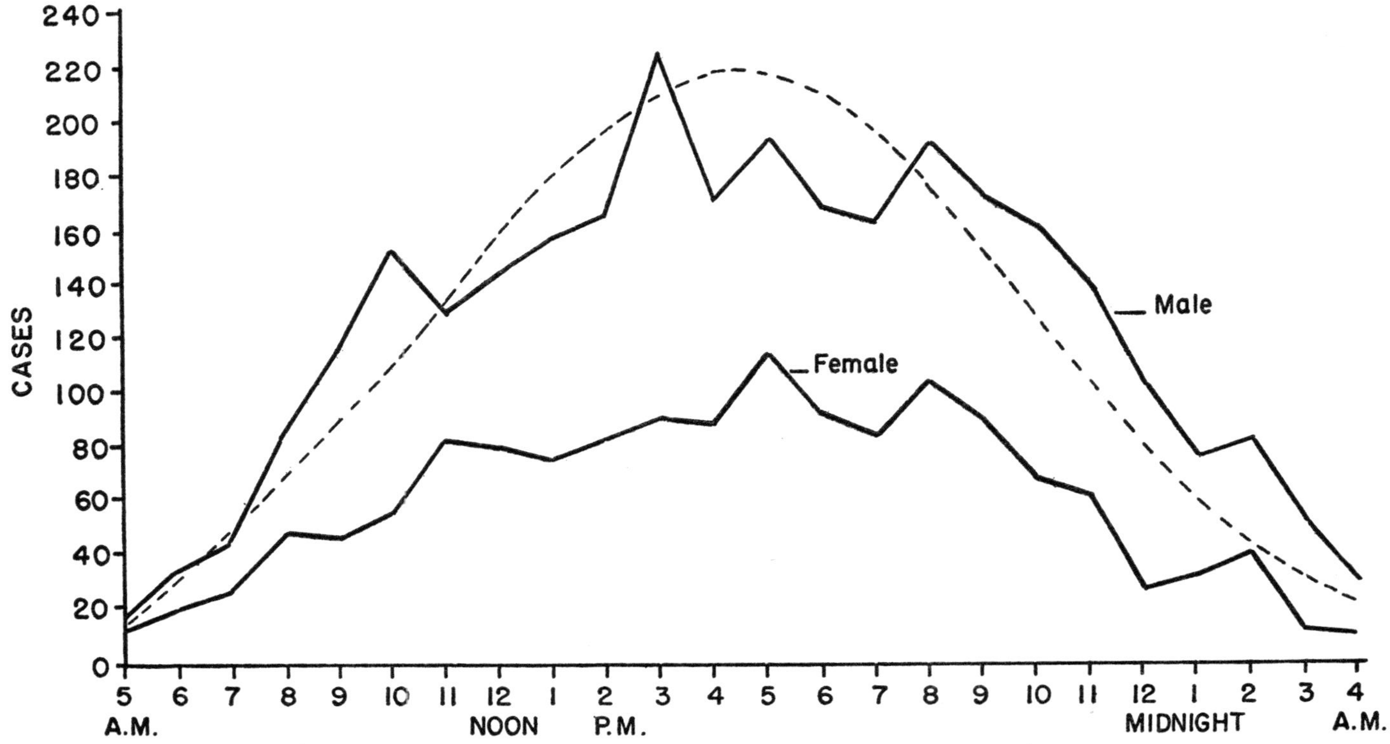

Chart 20
Percentage of Non-Industrial Accidents by Hour and Three Age Groups 1930-1948

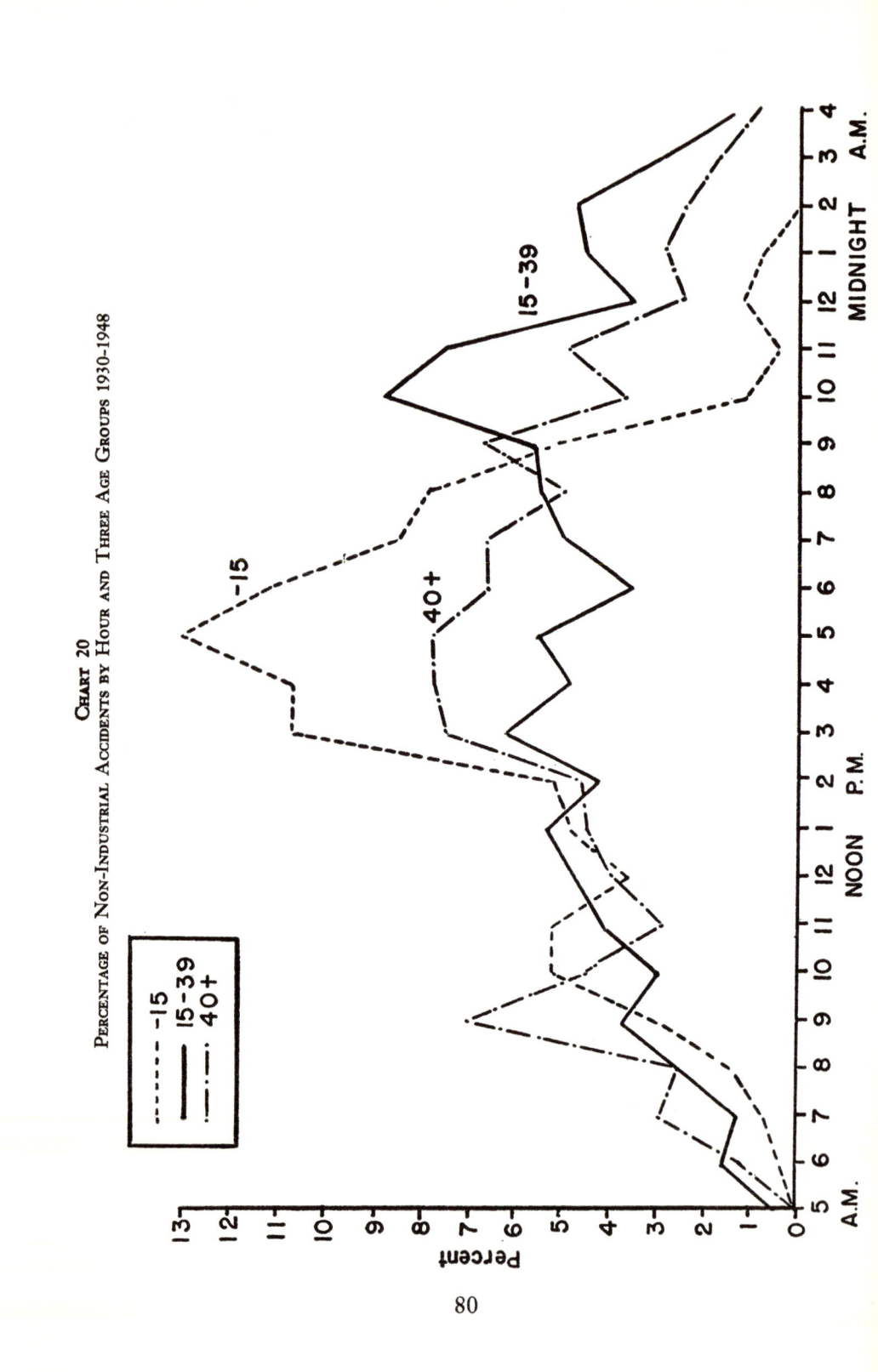

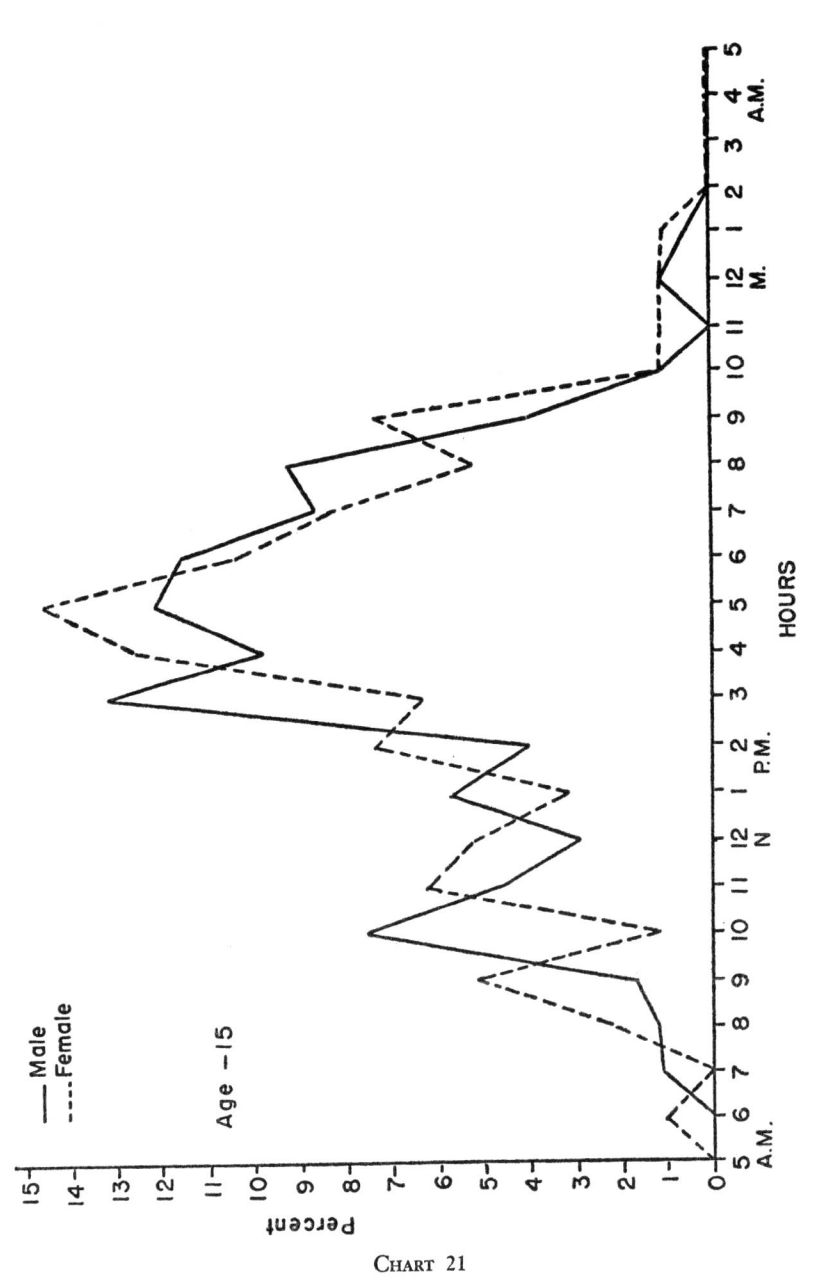

CHART 21

HOUR OF NON-INDUSTRIAL ACCIDENTS BY SEX, UNDER AGE OF FIFTEEN 1930-1948

CHART 22

Hour of Non-Industrial Accidents by Sex, Age 15-39, 1930-1948

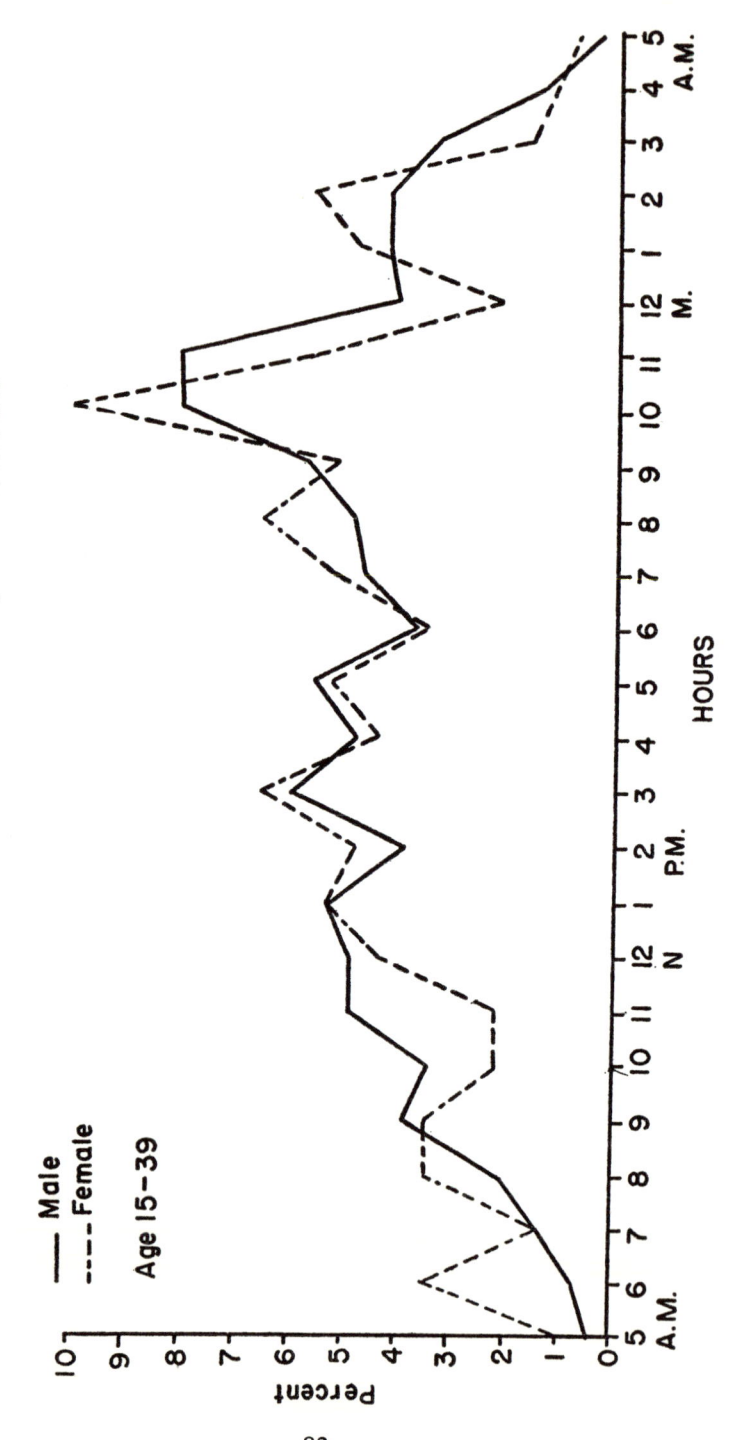

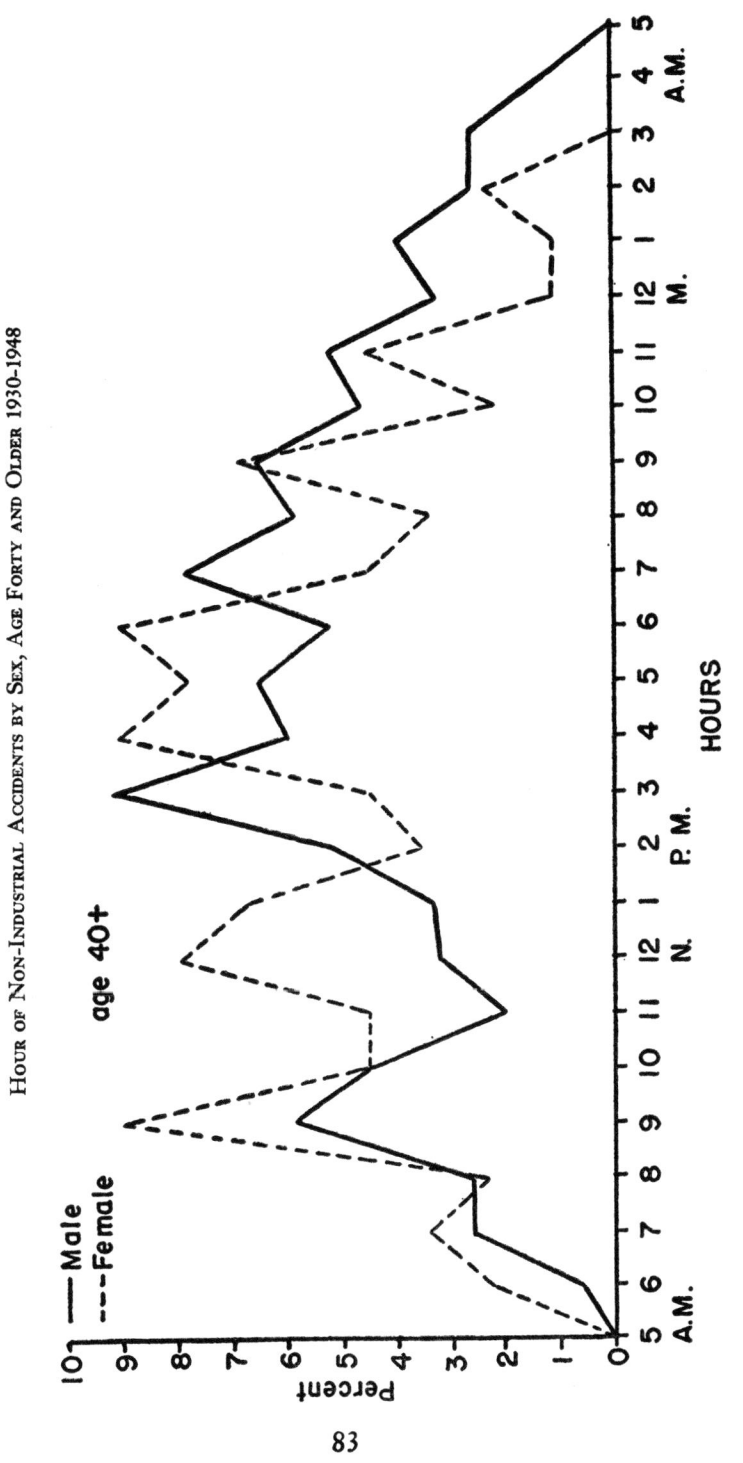

CHART 23

HOUR OF NON-INDUSTRIAL ACCIDENTS BY SEX, AGE FORTY AND OLDER 1930-1948

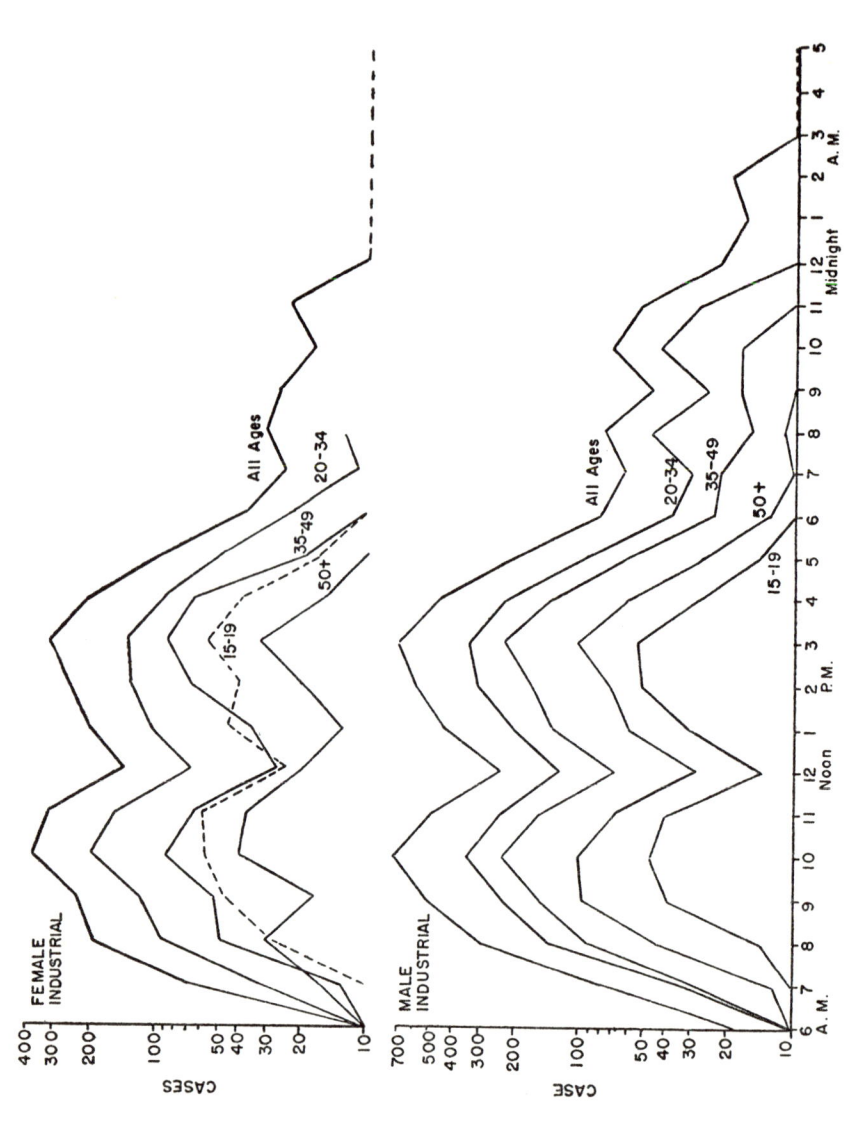

CHART 24

HOUR OF INDUSTRIAL ACCIDENTS BY SEX AND AGE 1947

CHART 25

PERCENTAGE OF INDUSTRIAL ACCIDENTS BY HOUR AND SEX (2105 CASES) 1947

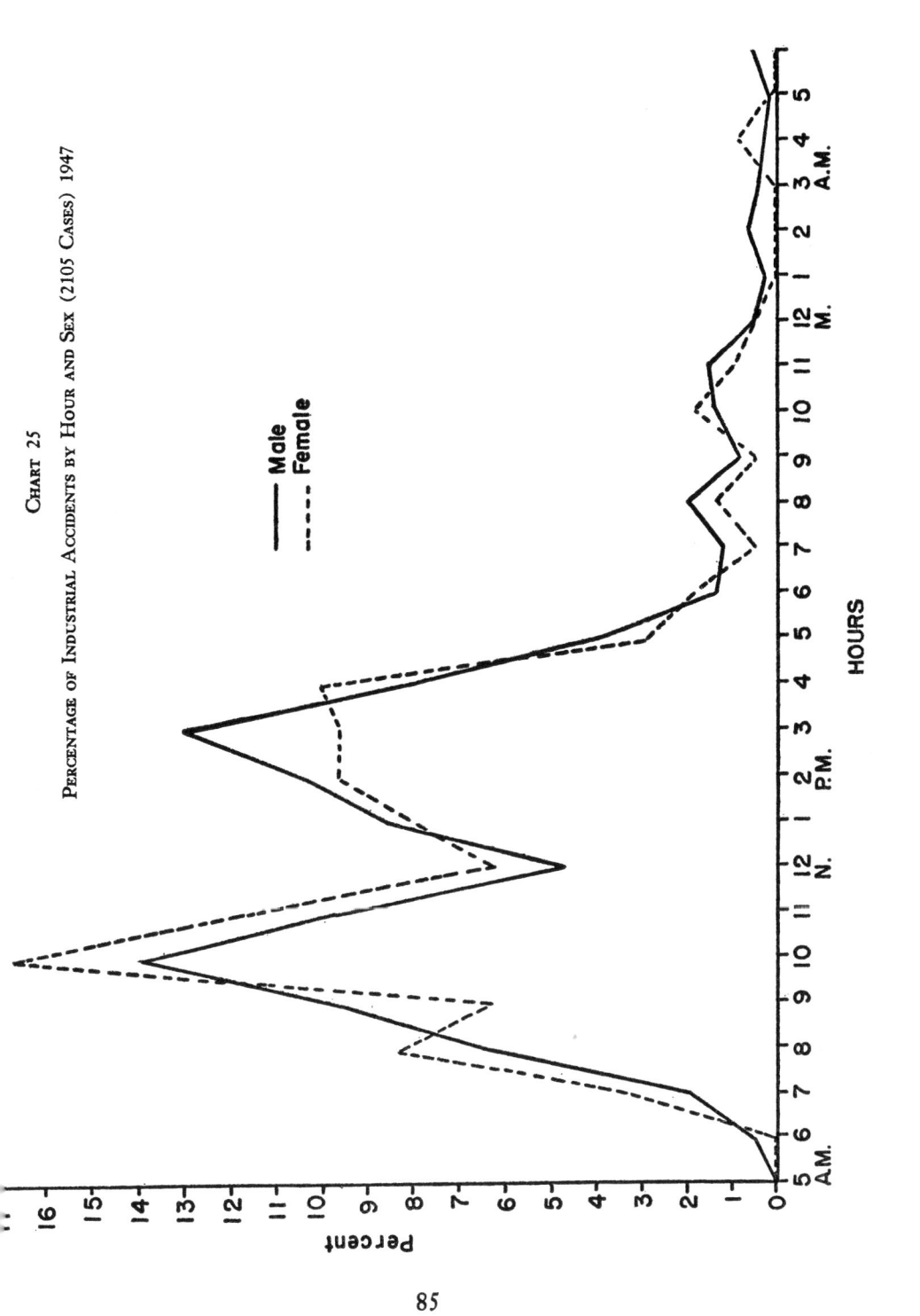

CHART 26

PERCENTAGE OF NON-INDUSTRIAL ACCIDENTS BY EIGHT THREE-HOUR INTERVALS BY AGE 1930-49
(DESIGNATED HOUR AT PEAK REPRESENTS MEDIAN)

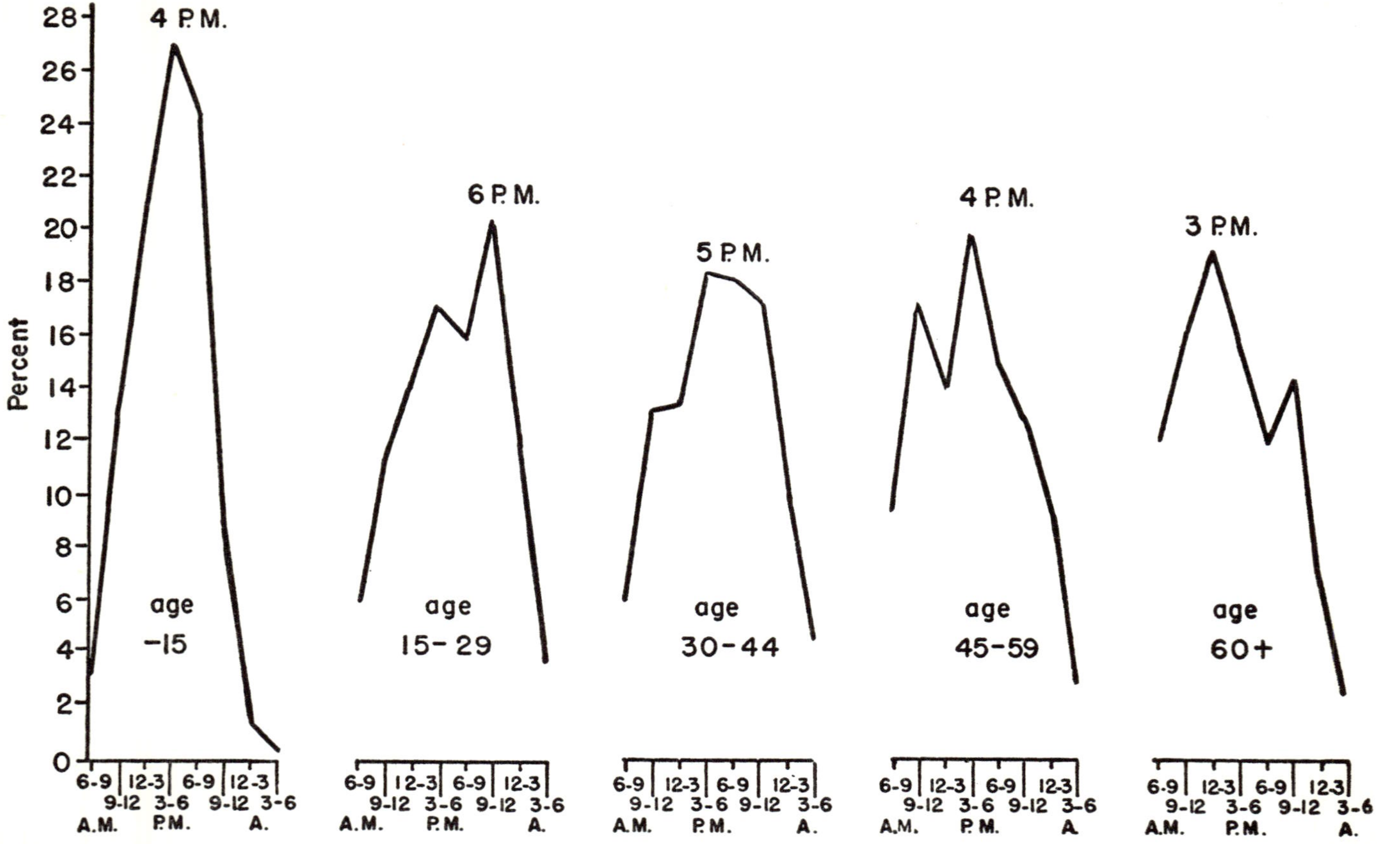

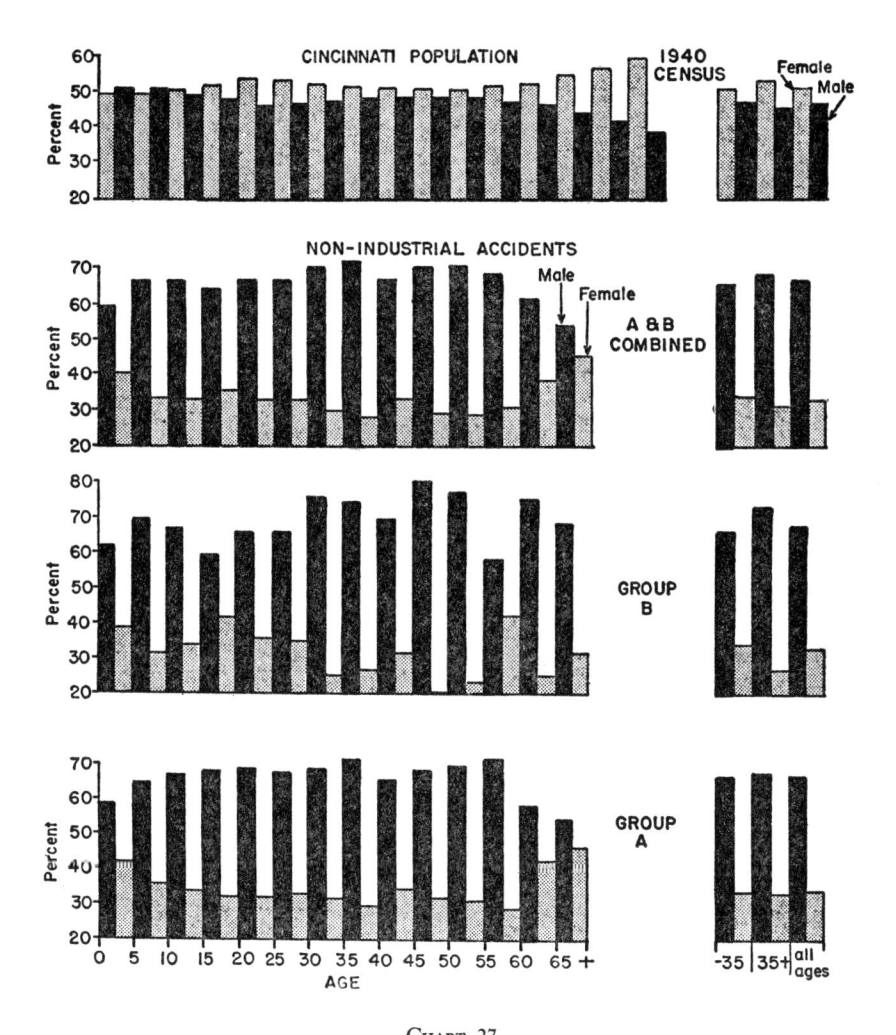

CHART 27

PERCENTAGE OF NON-INDUSTRIAL ACCIDENTS (1930-1948) BY AGE AND SEX
IN RELATION TO CINCINNATI'S POPULATION (1940)

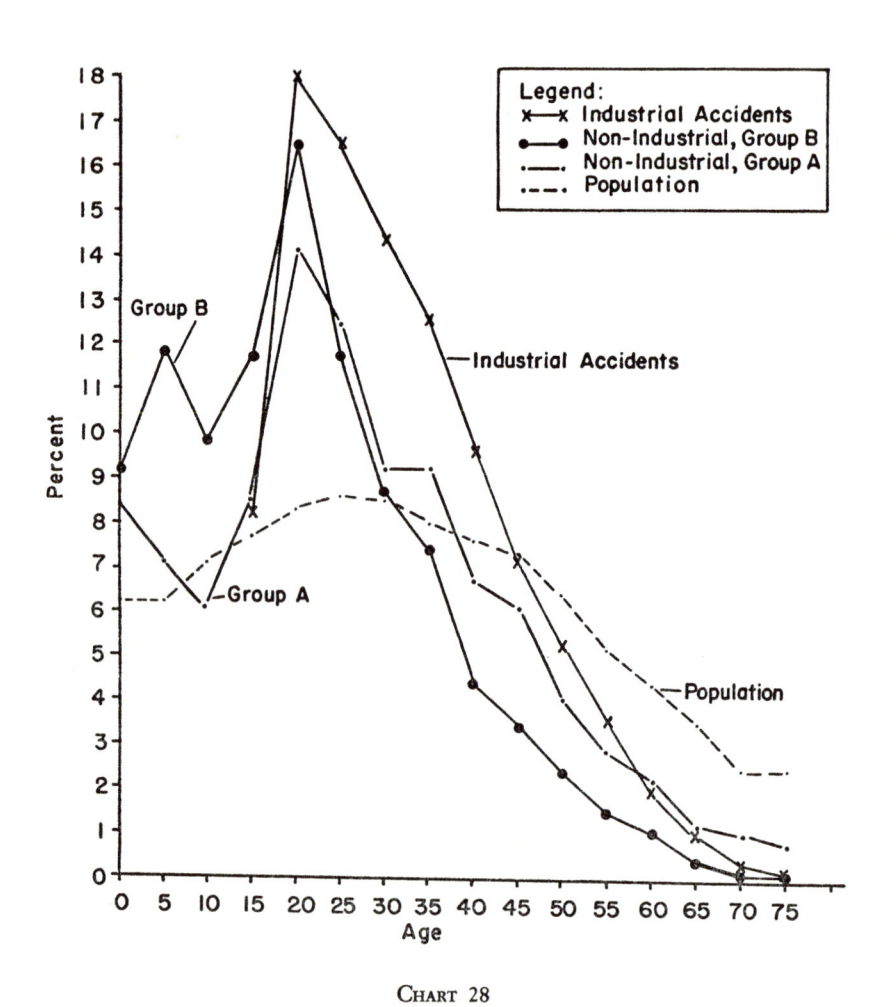

CHART 28

PERCENTAGE OF INDUSTRIAL AND NON-INDUSTRIAL ACCIDENTS (1930-1948) BY AGE IN RELATION TO CINCINNATI'S POPULATION (1940)

CHART 29

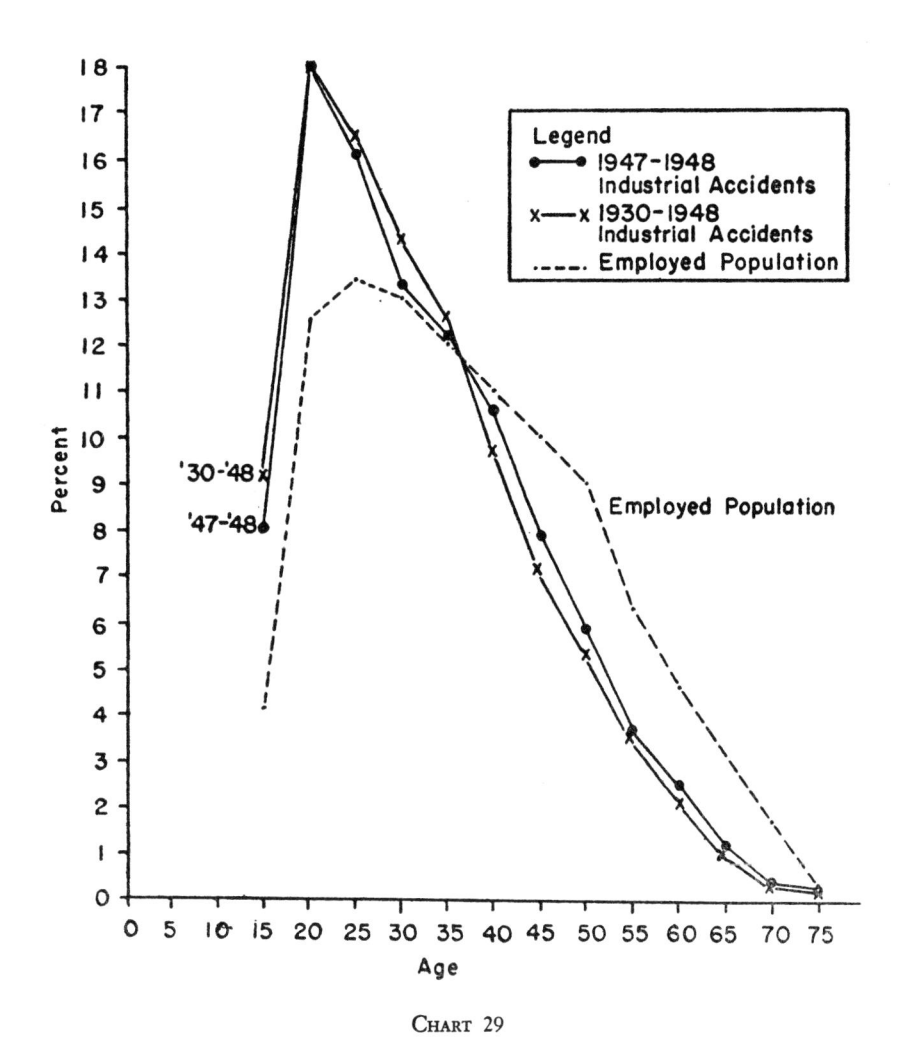

PERCENTAGE OF INDUSTRIAL ACCIDENTS (1930-1948), (1947-1948) BY AGE IN RELATION TO CINCINNATI'S EMPLOYED POPULATION (1946 U. S. SPECIAL CENSUS)

CHART 30

Non-Industrial Accidents (1930-1948) by Age and Sex

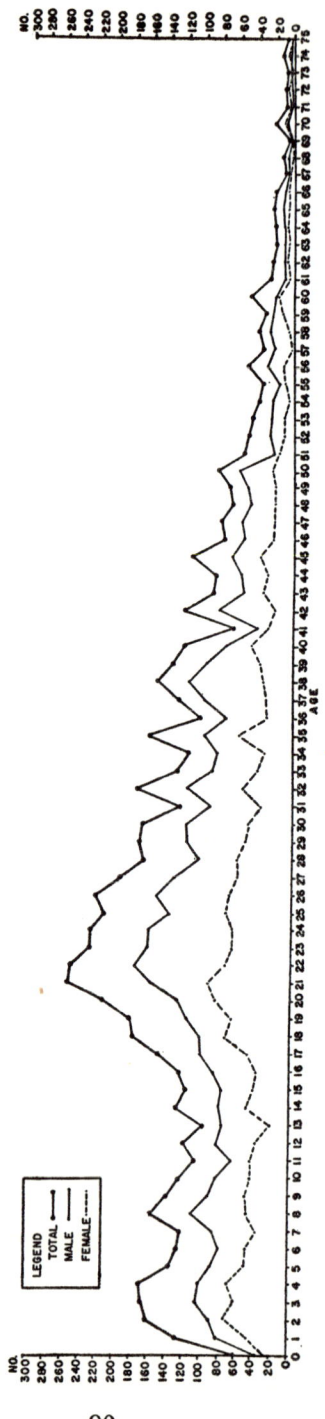

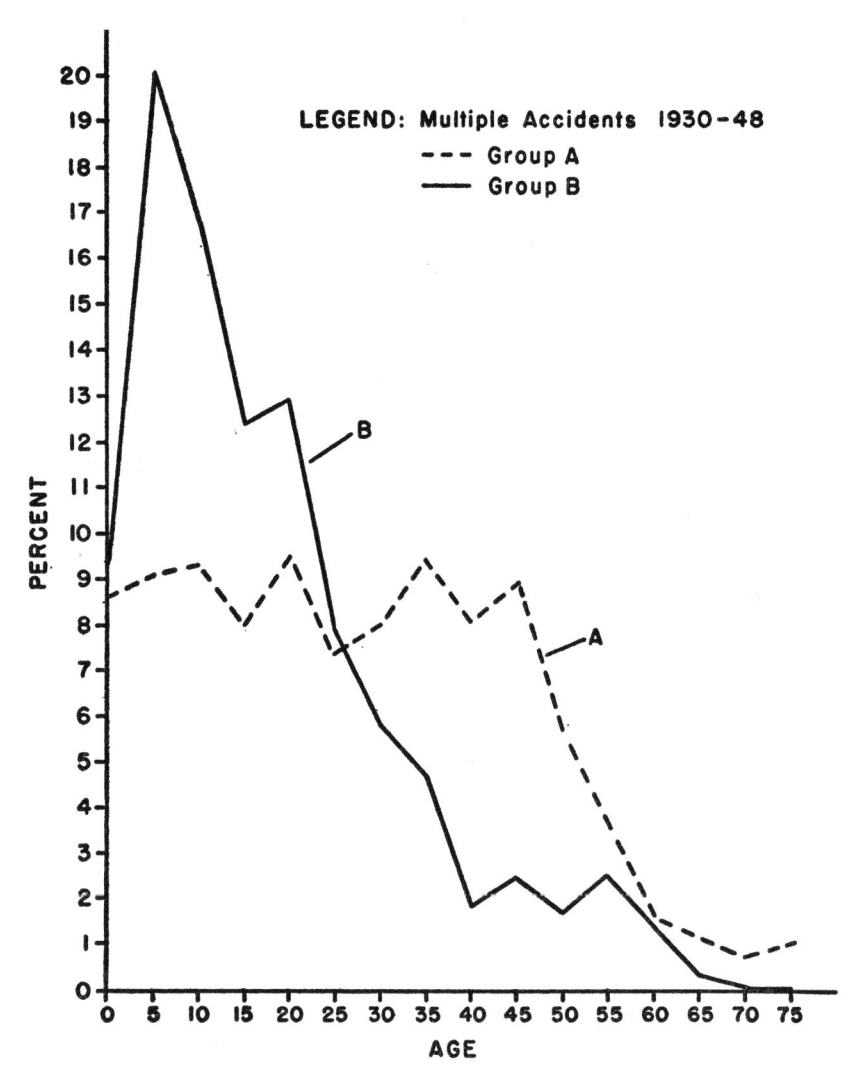

CHART 31

PERCENTAGE OF NON-INDUSTRIAL MULTIPLE ACCIDENTS
GROUPS A AND B BY AGE (1930-1948)

CHART 32

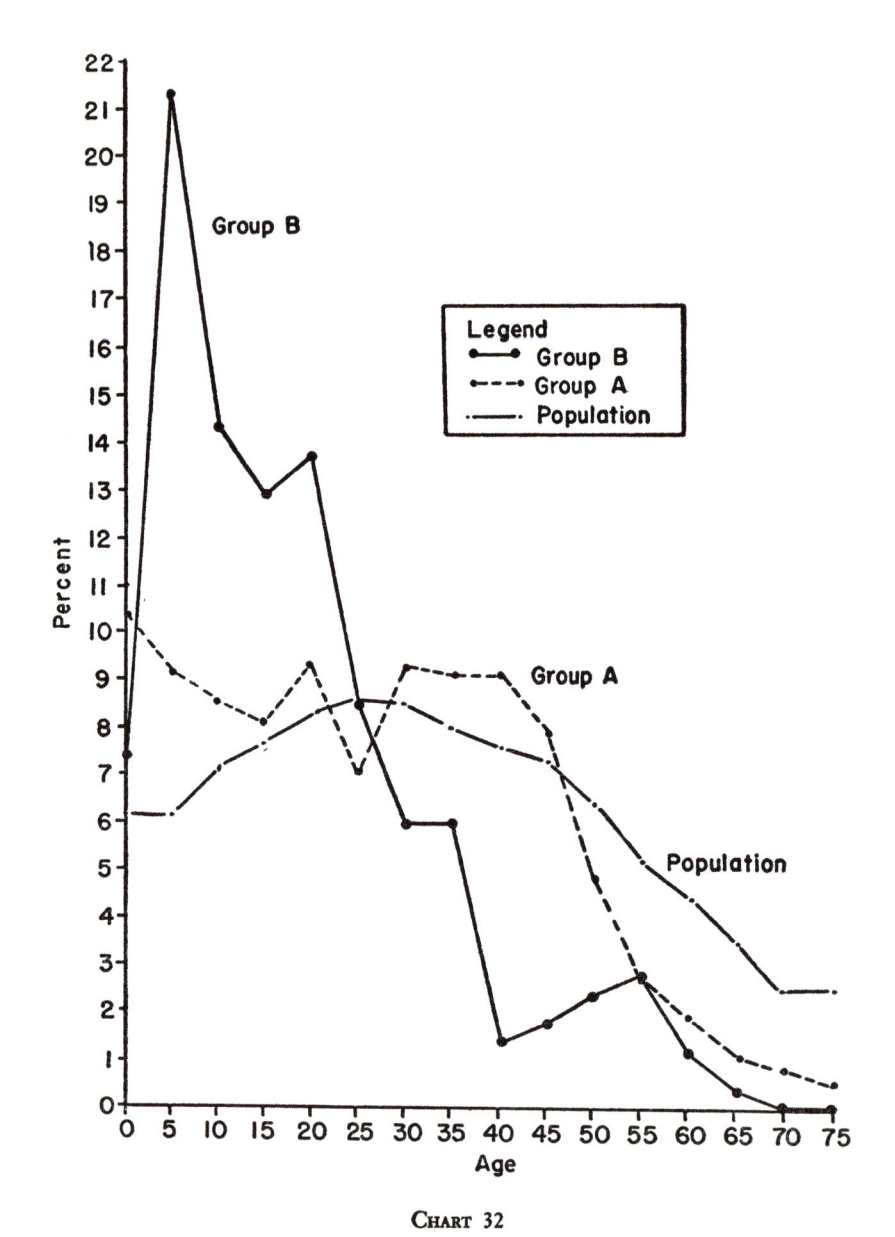

PERCENTAGE OF NON-INDUSTRIAL MULTIPLE ACCIDENTS GROUPS A AND B BY AGE
(1930-1941, 1942-1944, 1945 AND 1946-1948 COMBINED)

CHART 33

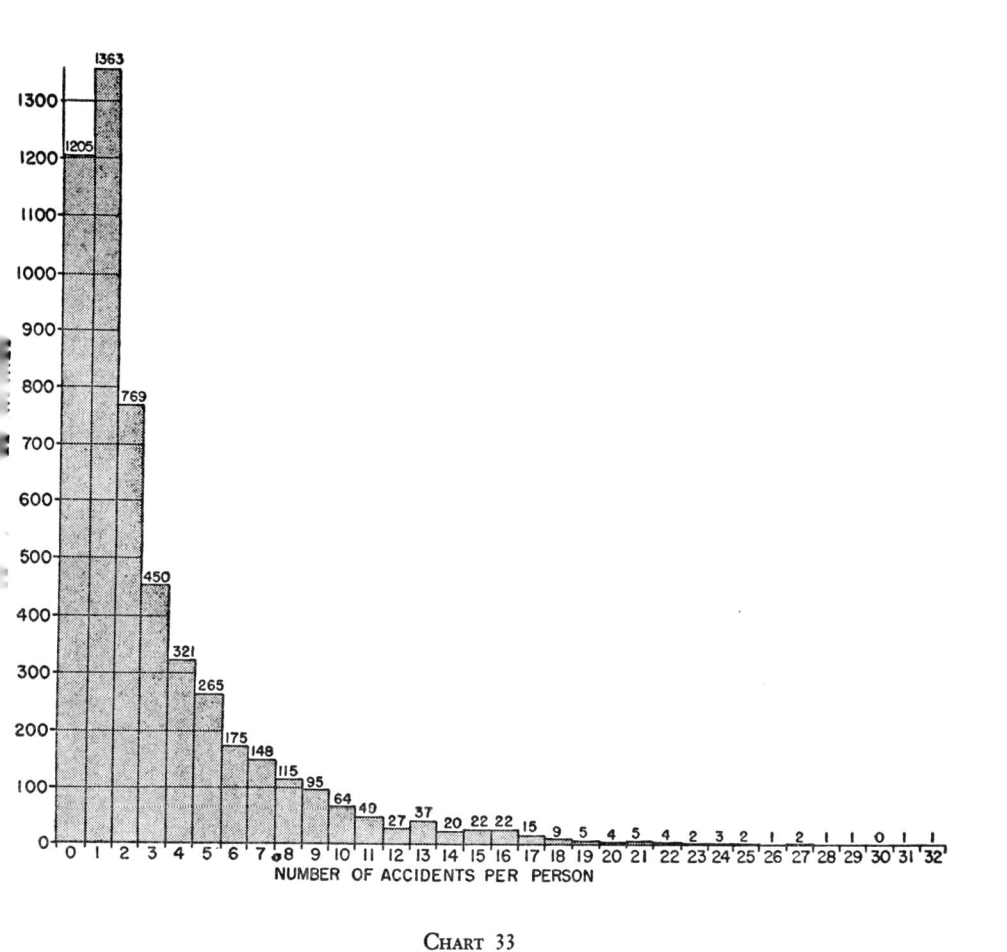

NUMBER OF PERSONS INJURED AND NUMBER OF ACCIDENTS PER PERSON IN 5208 WORKERS IN 1948
(64) (WOLFF)

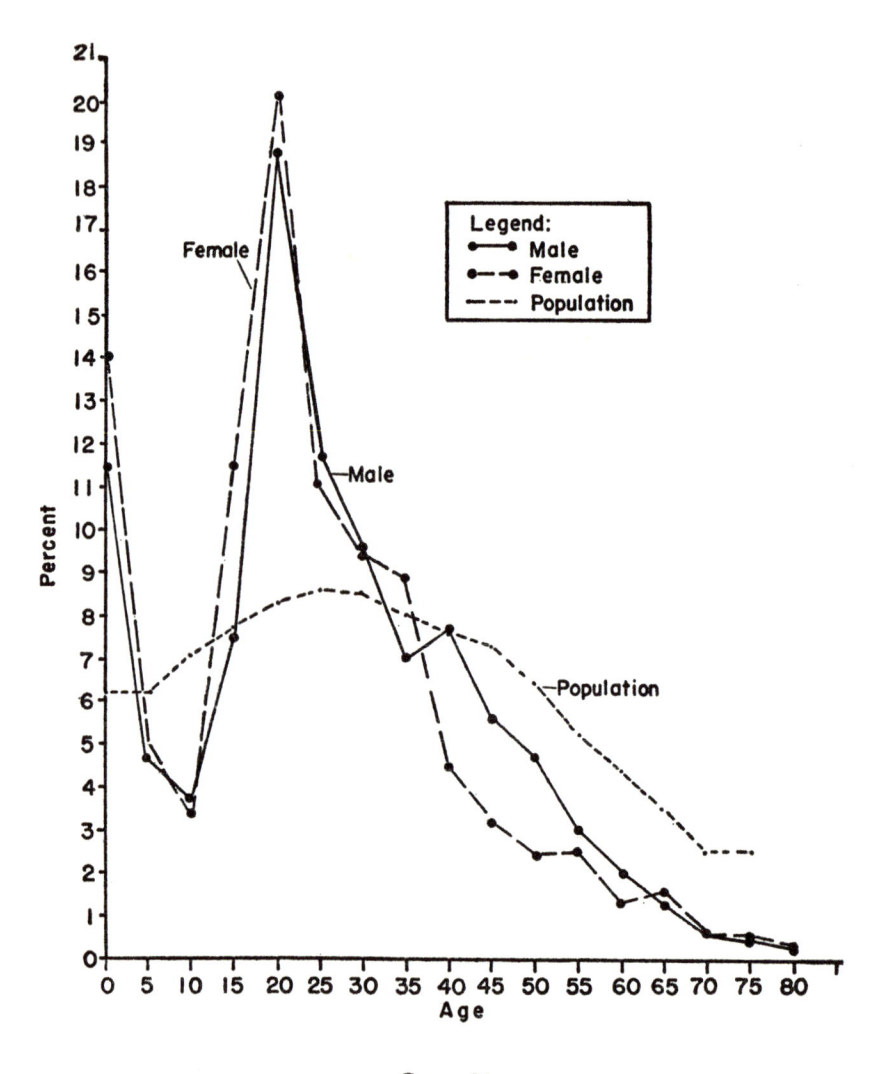

CHART 34

PERCENTAGE OF ILLNESS FROM ALL CAUSES BY AGE AND SEX, 1947-48; AND CINCINNATI'S POPULATION, 1940 CENSUS

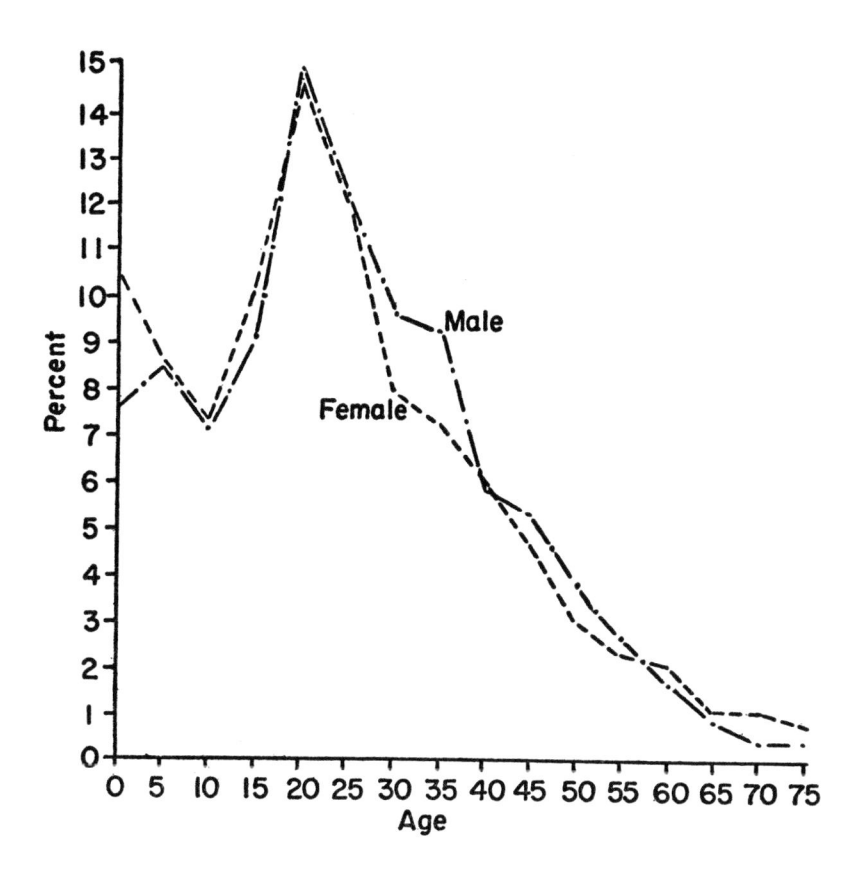

CHART 35

PERCENTAGE OF NON-INDUSTRIAL ACCIDENTS BY AGE AND SEX, 1930-1948

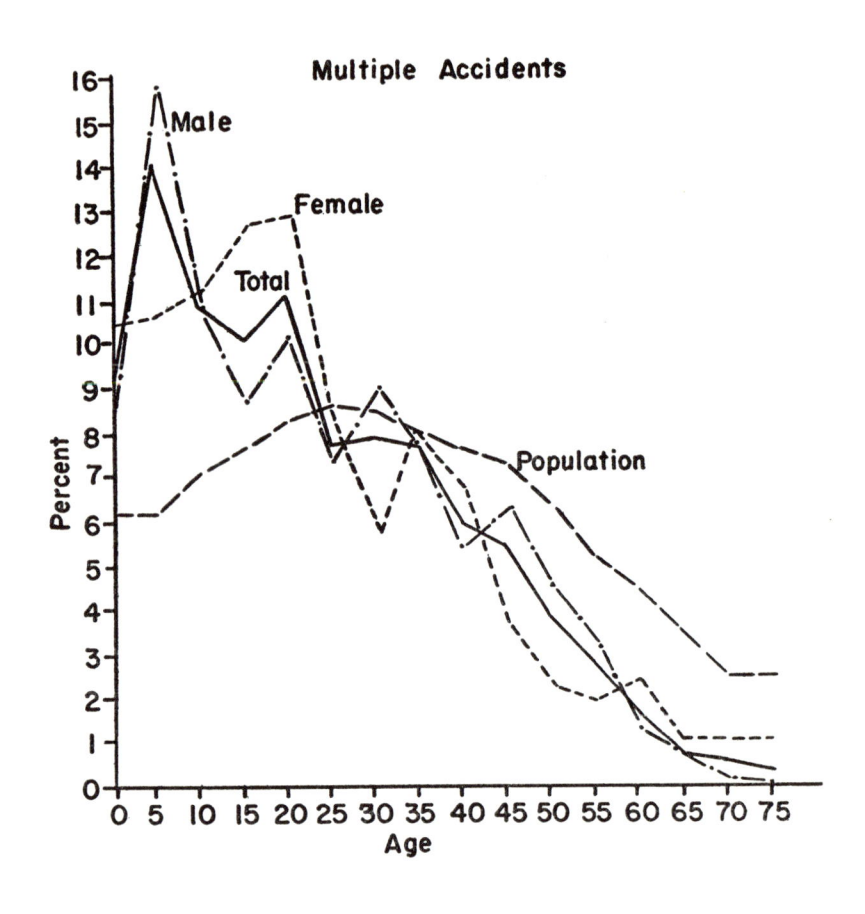

CHART 36

PERCENTAGE OF NON-INDUSTRIAL MULTIPLE ACCIDENTS BY AGE AND SEX, 1930-'41, 1942-'44, 1945 AND 1946-'48, COMBINED, IN RELATION TO CINCINNATI'S POPULATION (1940)

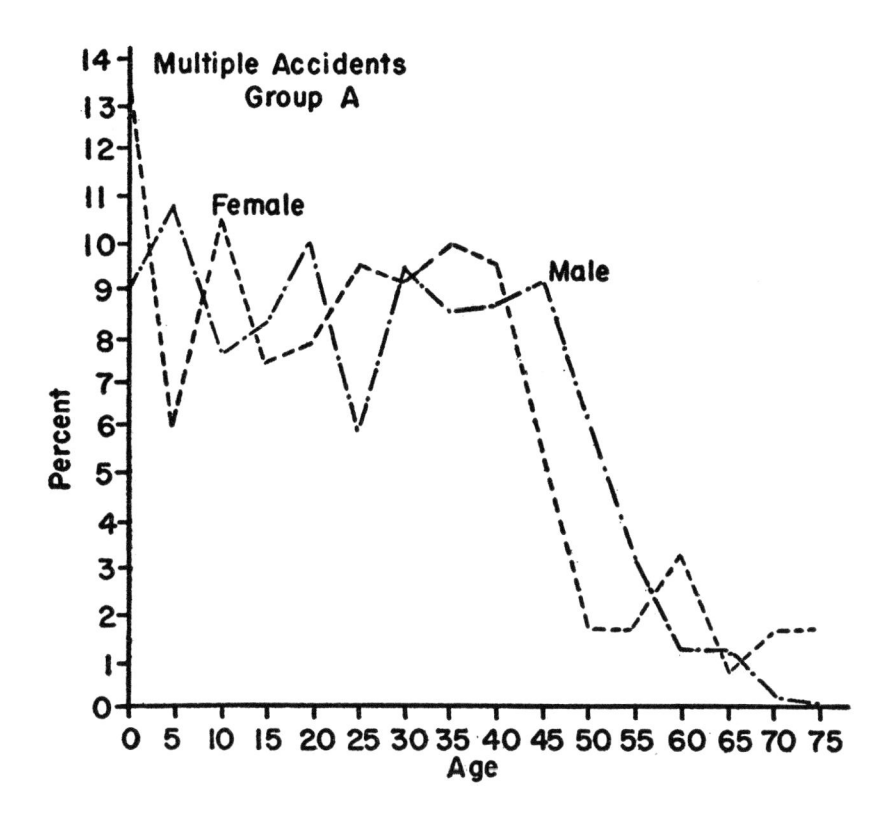

CHART 37

Percentage of Non-Industrial Multiple Accidents by Age and Sex, Group A, 1930-'41, 1942-'44, 1945 and 1946-'48, Combined

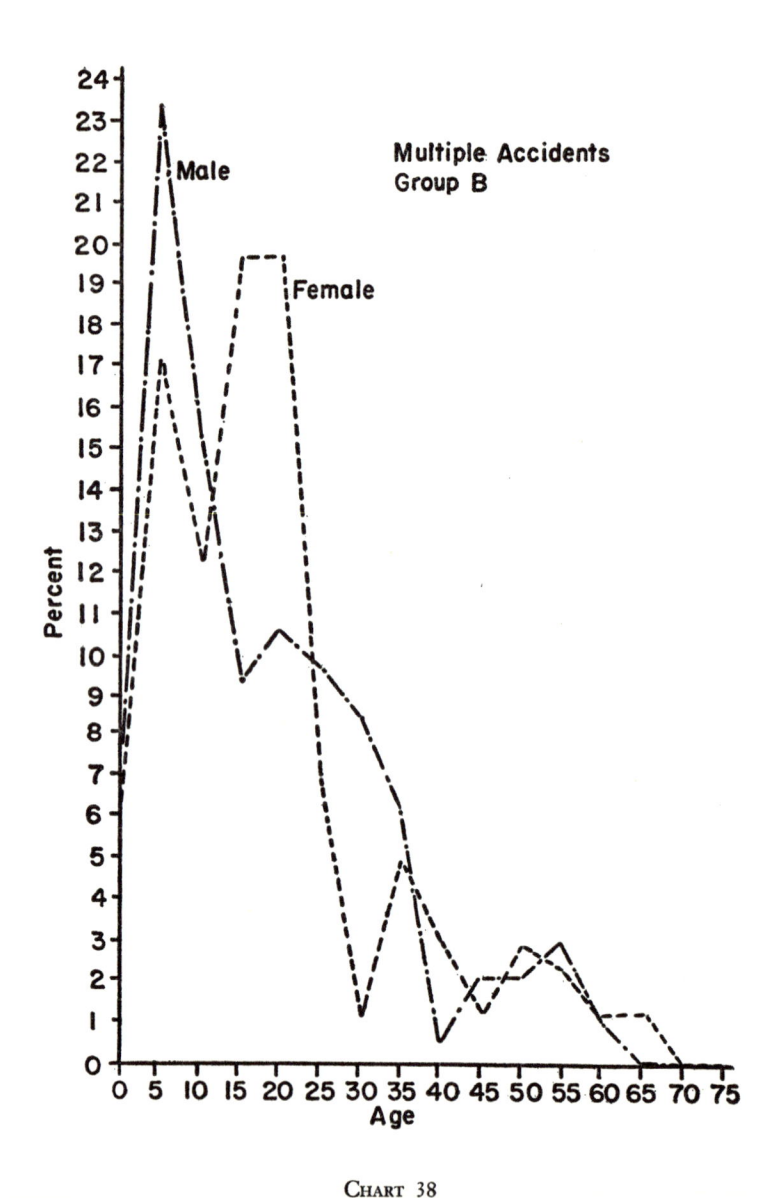

CHART 38

PERCENTAGE OF NON-INDUSTRIAL MULTIPLE ACCIDENTS BY AGE AND SEX, GROUP B, 1930-'41, 1942-'44, 1945 AND 1946-'48, COMBINED

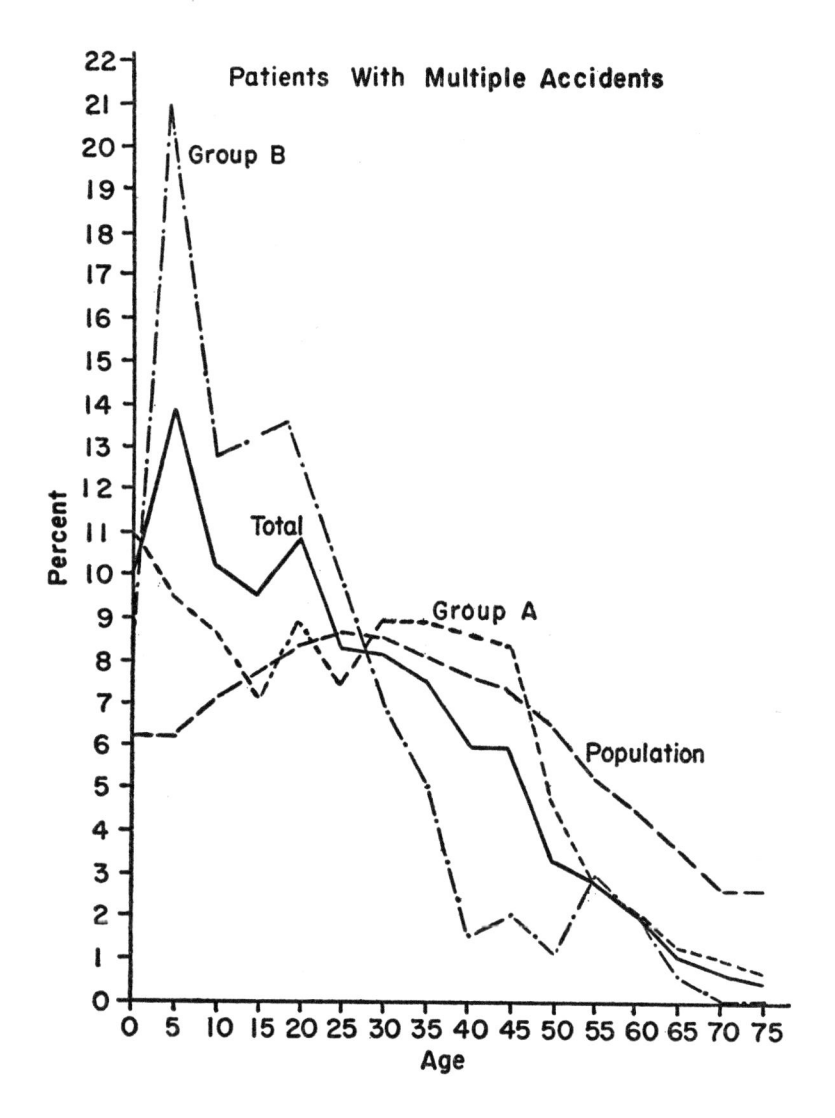

CHART 39

PERCENTAGE OF NON-INDUSTRIAL PATIENTS WITH MULTIPLE ACCIDENTS BY AGE, IN GROUPS A AND B, 1930-'41, 1942-'44, 1945 AND 1946-'48, COMBINED, IN RELATION TO CINCINNATI'S POPULATION (1940)

CHART 40

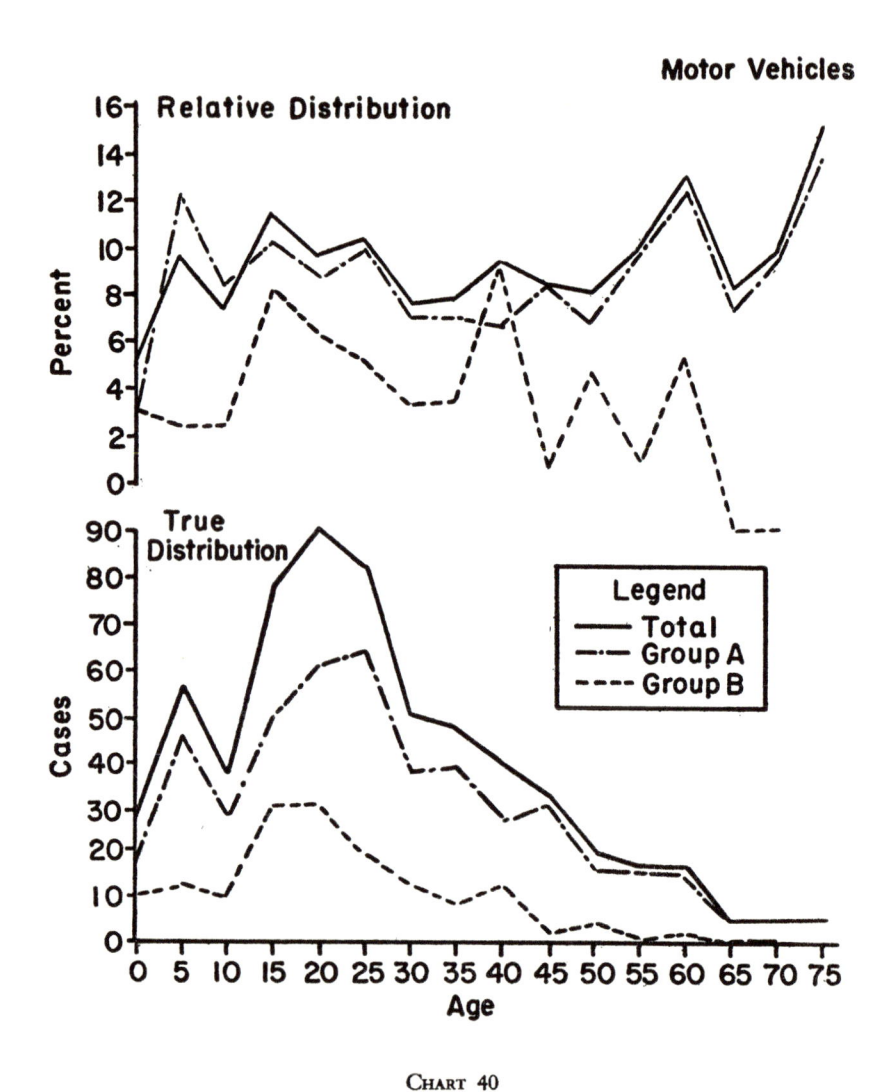

CASES FROM MOTOR VEHICLES AND THEIR RELATIVE DISTRIBUTION BY AGE, IN GROUPS A AND B, NON-INDUSTRIAL, 1930-1948

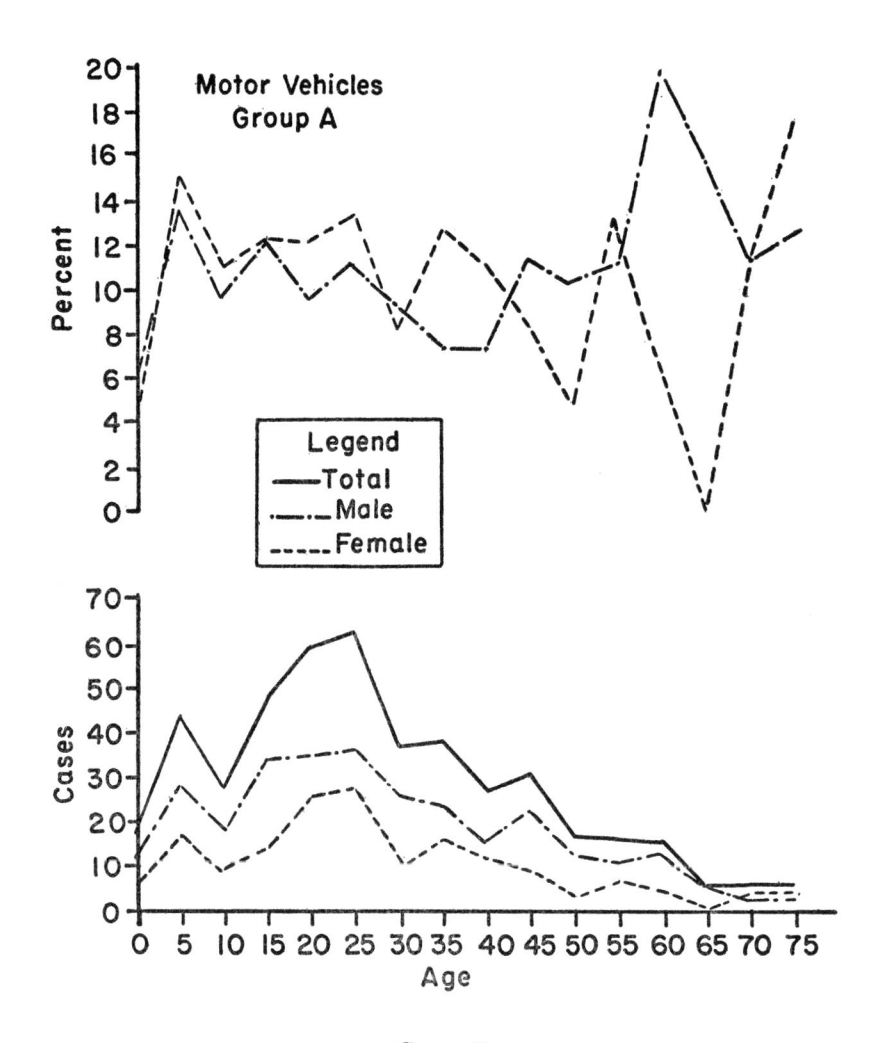

CHART 41

CASES FROM MOTOR VEHICLES AND THEIR RELATIVE DISTRIBUTION BY AGE AND SEX, GROUP A, NON-INDUSTRIAL, 1930-1948

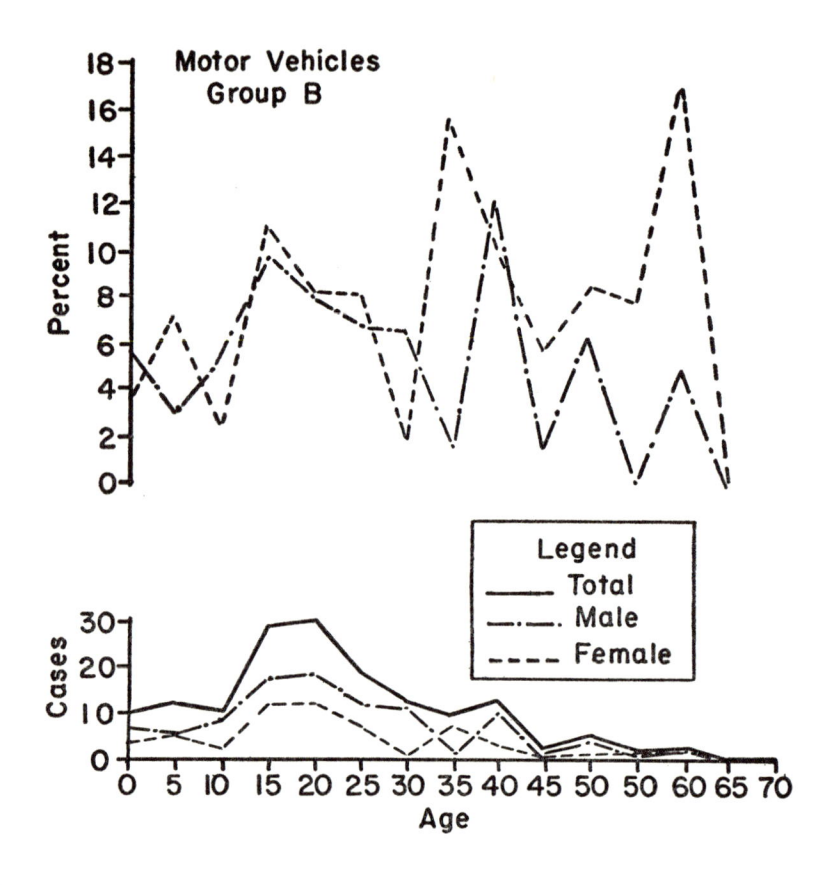

CHART 42

Cases from Motor Vehicles and Their Relative Distribution by Age and Sex, Group B, Non-Industrial, 1930-1948

CHART 43

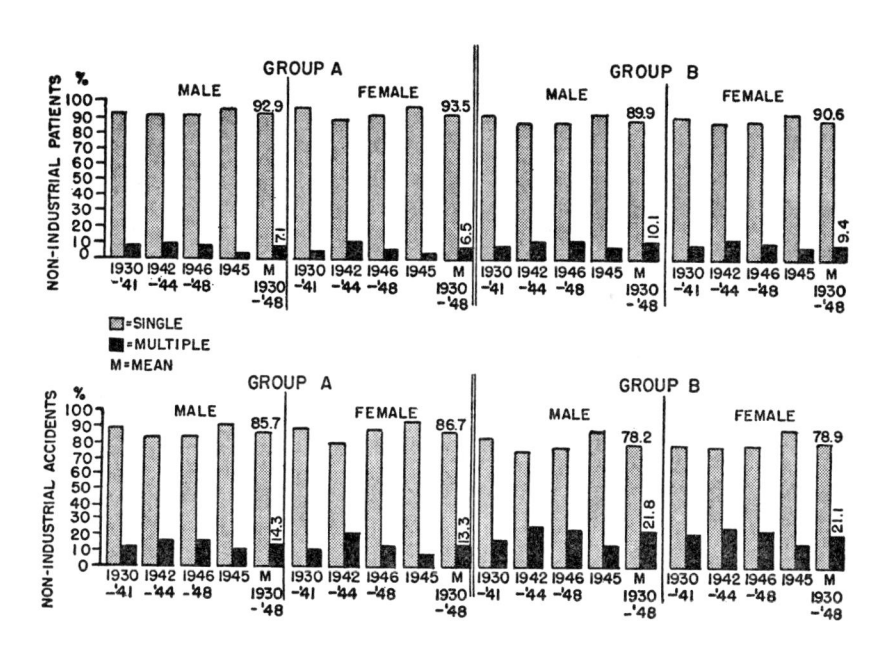

Per Cent Distribution of Single and Multiple Accidents in Non-Industrial Patients and Accidents, by Sex, in the Normally Adjusted (Group A) and in the Maladjusted (Group B) over a Nineteen-Year Period

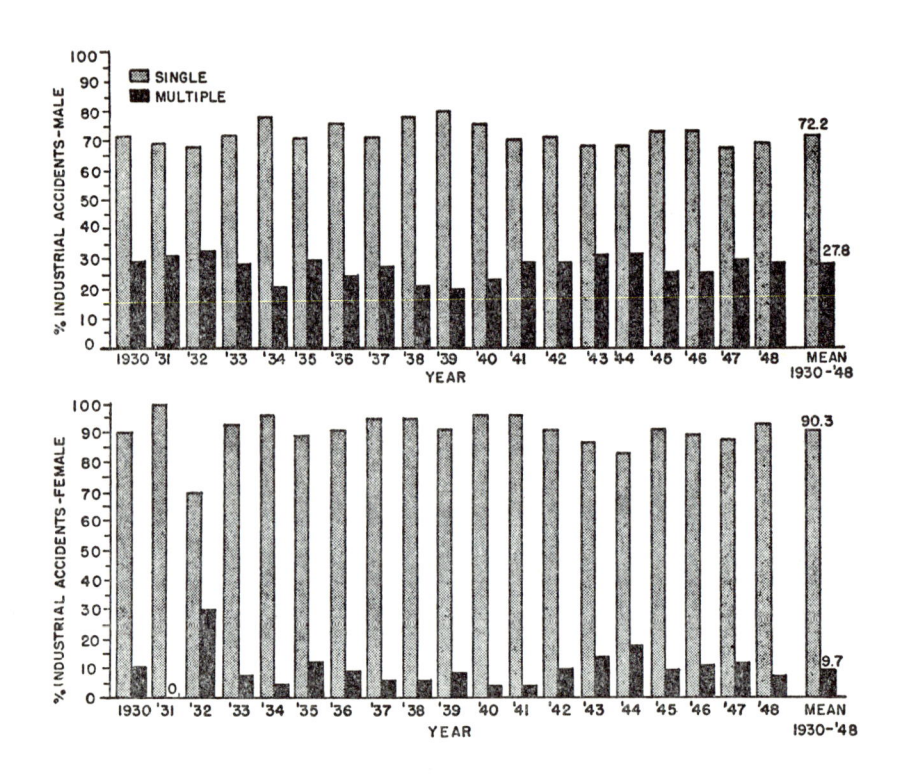

CHART 44

PER CENT DISTRIBUTION OF SINGLE AND MULTIPLE INDUSTRIAL ACCIDENTS BY SEX, OVER A NINETEEN-YEAR PERIOD

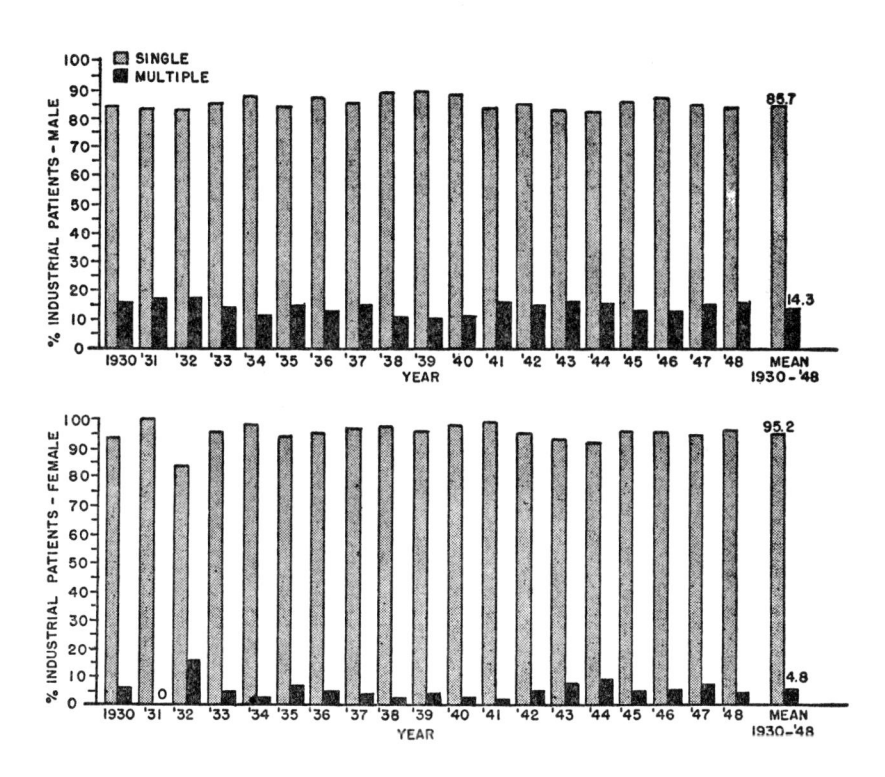

CHART 45

PER CENT DISTRIBUTION OF SINGLE AND MULTIPLE ACCIDENTS OF INDUSTRIAL PATIENTS BY SEX, OVER A NINETEEN-YEAR PERIOD

TABLE 1.1

INDUSTRIAL ACCIDENTS BY AGE AND SEX 1930–1948

Age	*Male Mult.	*Male Single	*Male Total	Female Mult.	Female Single	Female Total	*Male and Female Mult.	*Male and Female Single	*Male and Female Total	Number of Patients Male	Number of Patients Female	Number of Patients M and F
15–19	484	1562	2046	48	463	511	532	2025	2557	1596	487	2083
*20–24	*1237	*3154	*4391	76	561	637	*1313	*3715	*5028	*3232	597	*3829
25–29	1237	2902	4139	58	406	464	1295	3308	4603	2993	433	3426
30–34	1101	2596	3697	16	287	303	1117	2883	4000	2681	295	2976
35–39	955	2258	3213	20	277	297	975	2535	3510	2327	286	2613
40–44	685	1785	2470	30	204	234	715	1989	2704	1844	217	2061
45–49	521	1333	1854	16	141	157	537	1474	2011	1372	149	1521
50–54	317	1003	1320	7	139	146	324	1142	1466	1033	142	1175
55–59	200	726	926	7	77	84	207	803	1010	739	80	819
60–64	103	447	550	2	34	36	105	481	586	454	35	489
65–69	40	207	247	2	24	26	42	231	273	212	25	237
70–74	8	82	90	..	6	6	8	88	96	83	6	89
75†	12	22	34	..	2	2	12	24	36	22	2	24
15–75†	*6900	*18077	*24977	282	2621	2903	*7182	*20698	*27880	*18588	2754	*21342
			24382						27235	18180		20934

*Corrected for males in service or out of labor market, using 1947–48 as standard. The actual male accidents are 3,796 and male and female combined are 4,383, while the male patients number 2,824 and the male and female combined are 3,421. The actual grand totals for males of all ages and for males and females combined appear in the last line.

106

TABLE 1.2

NON-INDUSTRIAL ACCIDENTS BY AGE, SEX AND GROUPS A, B, AND A AND B 1930–1948

	Group A							Group B							Groups A & B						
	Number Accidents			Number Patients			Number Accidents			Number Patients			Number Accidents			Number Patients		
	M	F	M&F	M	F	M&F	M	F	M&F	M	F	M&F	M	F	M&F	M	F	M&F
0–4	266	189	455	243	173	416	133	86	219	119	80	199	399	275	674	362	253	615
5–9	245	137	382	218	129	347	198	89	287	152	71	223	443	226	669	370	200	570
10–14	216	111	327	195	98	293	171	83	254	126	69	195	387	194	581	321	167	488
15–19	315	152	467	291	141	432	176	122	298	160	100	260	491	274	765	451	241	692
20–24	438	241	679	410	231	641	222	143	365	202	122	324	660	384	1044	612	353	965
25–29	367	220	587	352	208	560	173	101	274	156	95	251	540	321	861	508	303	811
30–34	327	159	486	301	147	448	153	53	206	134	52	186	480	212	692	435	199	634
35–39	360	142	502	339	127	466	118	48	166	107	43	150	478	190	668	446	170	616
40–44	237	124	361	212	112	324	69	33	102	68	30	98	306	157	463	280	142	422
45–49	231	107	338	208	100	308	67	17	84	63	16	79	298	124	422	271	116	387
50–54	155	67	222	138	65	203	46	13	59	44	13	57	201	80	281	182	78	260
55–59	110	44	154	101	42	143	21	17	38	17	11	28	131	61	192	118	53	171
60–64	70	50	120	67	46	113	25	7	32	18	6	24	95	57	152	85	52	137
65–69	39	26	65	36	25	61	4	4	8	4	3	7	43	30	73	40	28	68
70–74	23	31	54	22	29	51	3	..	3	3	..	3	26	31	57	25	29	54
75 †	23	19	42	23	17	40	..	1	1	..	1	1	23	20	43	23	18	41
Total	3422	1819	5241	3156	1690	4846	1579	817	2396	1373	712	2085	5001	2636	7637	4529	2402	6931

107

Table 1.3

Non-Industrial Accidents by Age and Sex, Groups A and B 1946 - 1948

Group A

Age	Number Accidents M	Number Accidents F	Number Accidents M&F	Number Patients M	Number Patients F	Number Patients M&F
0-4	112	104	216	99	93	192
5-9	91	54	145	77	51	128
10-14	67	42	109	59	36	95
15-19	89	51	140	83	50	133
20-24	205	98	303	190	95	285
25-29	181	101	282	171	98	269
30-34	126	73	199	115	65	180
35-39	139	62	201	127	57	184
40-44	67	46	113	62	43	105
45-49	63	47	110	55	43	98
50-54	54	25	79	47	25	72
55-59	28	25	53	27	23	50
60-64	31	14	45	31	14	45
65-69	12	13	25	12	13	25
70-74	11	14	25	10	13	23
75†	10	6	16	10	6	16
Total	1286	775	2061	1175	725	1900

Group B

Age	Number Accidents M	Number Accidents F	Number Accidents M&F	Number Patients M	Number Patients F	Number Patients M&F
0-4	54	29	83	47	29	76
5-9	59	31	90	45	26	71
10-14	62	22	84	44	20	64
15-19	57	48	105	51	39	90
20-24	112	67	179	101	52	153
25-29	74	44	118	62	41	103
30-34	64	21	85	58	21	79
35-39	58	18	76	52	17	69
40-44	31	11	42	30	11	41
45-49	26	9	35	23	8	31
50-54	20	2	22	20	2	22
55-59	10	13	23	7	7	14
60-64	8	3	11	7	2	9
65-69	2	1	3	2	1	3
70-74	1	..	1	1	..	1
75†	..	1	1	..	1	1
Total	638	320	958	550	277	827

TABLE 1.4
PRINCIPAL CLASSES OF ACCIDENTS IN 1951
(71) (National Safety Council)

Classes	Total Deaths	Rate	Disabling Injuries
Motor vehicles	37,300	24.3	1,350,000
Home	28,000	18.3	4,250,000
Occupation	16,000	10.4	2,100,000
Public (Non-motor) (Vehicle)	15,000	9.8	1,900,000
Total	96,300		9,600,000

TABLE 1.5
PRINCIPAL TYPES OR MEANS OF ACCIDENTS IN 1951
(71) (National Safety Council)

Types	Total Deaths	Rate
1. Motor-vehicles	37,300	24.3
2. Falls	20,600	13.4
3. Drownings	6,500	4.2
4. Fire, burns	6,500	4.2
5. Railroad	3,550	2.3
6. Firearms	2,250	1.5
7. Poison gases	1,650	1.1
8. Poisons (other)	1,500	1.0
9. All other types	17,200	10.8
TOTAL	97,050	

TABLE 1.6
PRINCIPAL CLASSES OF ACCIDENTS AMONG WORKERS IN 1951
(71) (National Safety Council)

Classes	Deaths	Injuries
All accidents	49,000	4,600,000
1. At work	16,000	2,100,000
2. Away from work	33,000	2,500,000
a. Motor vehicle	19,800	700,000
b. Public non-motor vehicle	7,500	950,000
c. Home	5,700	850,000

TABLE 2.1

Types of Injury in Industrial Accidents by Sex and by Two Age Groups 1947

Nature of Injury	Sex	Under 35 Male	Under 35 Female	Under 35 Total	35 and Older Male	35 and Older Female	35 and Older Total	Total All Ages Male	Total All Ages Female	Total All Ages Total
1. Lacerations		353	44	397	293	35	328	646	79	725
2. Contusions		381	34	415	324	37	361	705	71	776
3. Abrasions and friction burns		68	3	71	44	5	49	112	8	120
4. Fractures		59	7	66	87	8	95	146	15	161
5. Foreign body in eye		190	15	205	135	8	143	325	23	348
6. Puncture wounds		95	32	127	72	15	87	167	47	214
7. Sprains (joints)		43	7	50	36	5	41	79	12	91
8. Strains (muscle and ligament)		92	8	100	84	4	88	176	12	188
9. Burns		59	13	72	40	6	46	99	19	118
10. Animal and human bites		7	....	7	3	....	3	10	....	10
11. Foreign body in body orifice		2	....	2	....	....	....	2	....	2
12. Contact dermatitis		8	3	11	6	1	7	14	4	18
13. Dislocations		2	....	2	3	....	3	5	....	5
14. Severed tendons		20	....	20	17	1	18	37	1	38
15. Amputations		8	2	10	11	....	11	19	2	21
16. Poisonings		3	....	3	....	....	....	3	....	3
Total Cases		1390	168	1558	1155	125	1280	2545	293	2838

TABLE 2.2
TYPES OF INJURY IN INDUSTRIAL ACCIDENTS BY SEX AND BY FIVE-YEAR AGE GROUPS 1947

Cases

Age	15–19			20–24			25–29			30–34			35–39			40–44			45–49			50–54			55–59			60–64			65–69			70†		
Sex	M	F	T	M	F	T	M	F	T	M	F	T	M	F	T	M	F	T	M	F	T	M	F	T	M	F	T	M	F	T	M	F	T	M	F	T
1. Laceration	62	12	74	120	18	138	92	10	102	79	4	83	83	14	97	64	7	71	48	6	54	40	3	43	25	2	27	18	2	20	12	1	13	3	..	3
2. Contusion	52	6	58	126	17	143	120	4	124	83	7	90	83	1	84	78	11	89	60	10	70	41	7	48	20	4	24	26	3	29	11	1	12	5	..	5
3. Abrasion and friction	3	..	3	28	2	30	18	1	19	19	..	19	14	..	14	5	1	6	5	..	5	7	2	9	8	..	8	5	..	5	1	..	1	..	..	..
4. Fracture	6	1	7	14	5	19	25	..	25	14	1	15	20	2	22	17	2	19	16	1	17	14	..	14	6	..	6	6	2	8	7	..	7	1	..	1
5. Foreign body in eye	22	4	26	47	4	51	64	5	69	57	2	59	52	6	58	35	2	37	22	..	22	12	..	12	9	..	9	1	..	1	4	..	4	..	..	..
6. Puncture wound	16	11	27	37	11	48	25	4	29	17	6	23	13	..	13	13	8	21	19	1	20	9	2	11	10	1	11	3	1	4	4	2	6	1	..	1
7. Sprain	6	1	7	14	2	16	13	3	16	10	1	11	11	2	13	5	2	7	9	..	9	7	1	8	3	..	3	3	..	3	..	..	..	..	..	..
8. Strain	7	..	7	32	6	38	25	1	26	28	1	29	27	2	29	16	1	17	14	..	14	16	1	17	3	..	3	3	..	3	2	..	2	3	..	3
9. Burn	10	1	11	14	4	18	18	4	22	17	4	21	15	..	15	3	1	4	7	4	11	7	..	7	4	..	4	3	..	3	1	..	1	1	..	1
10. Animal and human bites	1	..	1	3	..	3	2	..	2	1	..	1	1	..	1	..	..	..	1	..	1	1	..	1	1	..	1	..	..	..	..	..	..	..	..	..
11. Foreign body in body orifice	1	..	1	..	..	..	1	..	1	..	1	1	..	..	..	..	..	..	..	..	..	..	..	..	..	1	1	..	..	..	..	..	..	..	..	..
12. Contact dermatitis	1	..	1	2	1	3	4	1	5	1	1	2	..	..	..	1	..	1	2	1	3	2	..	2	2	..	2	..	..	..	..	..	..	..	..	..
13. Dislocation	..	..	..	..	..	..	2	..	2	..	..	..	1	..	1	..	..	..	1	..	1	1	..	1	..	..	..	..	..	..	..	..	..	..	..	..
14. Severed tendon	3	..	3	7	..	7	7	..	7	3	..	3	3	1	4	6	..	6	4	..	4	..	..	..	..	..	..	..	..	..	2	..	2	..	..	..
15. Amputation	1	1	2	4	1	5	3	..	3	..	..	..	2	..	2	5	..	5	..	..	..	..	..	..	..	..	..	..	..	..	1	..	1	..	..	..
16. Poisoning	..	..	..	..	..	..	..	..	..	..	..	..	..	..	..	..	..	..	..	..	..	..	..	..	..	..	..	..	..	..	..	..	..	..	..	..
Total No. Injuries	191	37	228	448	71	519	419	33	452	329	27	356	325	29	354	248	35	283	208	23	231	157	18	175	92	7	99	67	8	75	43	5	48	15	..	15

111

TABLE 2.3

TYPES OF INJURY IN NON-INDUSTRIAL ACCIDENTS BY AGE, SEX, AND GROUPS A AND B 1946-1948

	Under 35 Years						Number of Injuries 35 Years and Older						All Ages					
	A			B			A			B			A			B		
	M	F	T	M	F	T	M	F	T	M	F	T	M	F	T	M	F	T
1. Laceration	308	133	441	167	68	235	103	47	150	58	14	72	411	180	591	225	82	307
2. Contusion	247	119	366	157	77	234	112	63	175	58	36	94	359	182	541	215	113	328
3. Abrasion and friction	62	29	91	26	25	51	31	18	49	7	7	14	93	47	140	33	32	65
4. Fractures	52	22	74	43	12	55	39	22	61	12	11	23	91	44	135	55	23	78
5. Foreign body in eye	56	30	86	15	5	20	41	18	59	9	3	12	97	48	145	24	8	32
6. Puncture wound	24	16	40	15	12	27	17	5	22	10	1	11	41	21	62	25	13	38
7. Sprains	25	24	49	9	5	14	12	12	24	5	5	10	37	36	73	14	10	24
8. Strains	25	14	39	13	2	15	10	14	24	9	3	12	35	28	63	22	5	27
9. Burns	26	20	46	14	11	25	5	4	9	6	3	9	31	24	55	20	14	34
10. Animal and human bites	27	12	39	20	6	26	2	4	6	3	.	3	29	16	45	23	6	29
11. Foreign body in body orifice	8	5	13	1	4	5	2	5	7	1	1	2	10	10	20	2	5	7
12. Contact dermatitis	7	3	10	4	2	6	4	2	6	2	.	2	11	5	16	6	2	8
13. Dislocation	7	2	9	4	4	8	4	2	6	3	1	4	11	4	15	7	5	12
14. Severed tendon	3	2	5	2	1	3	1	.	1	3	.	3	4	2	6	5	1	6
15. Amputation	2	2	4	1	.	1	.	2	2	.	.	.	2	4	6	1	.	1
16. Poisoning	1	2	3	1	1	2	.	.	.	.	.	.	1	2	3	.	1	2
	880	435	1315	492	235	727	383	218	601	186	85	271	1263	653	1916	678	320	998

112

TABLE 3.1

PARTS OF BODY INJURED IN INDUSTRIAL ACCIDENTS BY AGE AND SEX* 1947

			Number of Anatomical Units
	Age	colspan=3	Under 35	colspan=3	35 and Older	colspan=3	Total All Ages
Anatomical Units Injured	Sex	M	F	T	M	F	T	M	F	T
1. Fingers		351	70	421	291	49	340	642	119	761
2. Eyes		223	16	239	153	5	158	376	21	397
3. Hands		95	18	113	86	8	94	181	26	207
4. Back (Lumbar)		57	6	63	60	5	65	117	11	128
5. Foot		63	6	69	47	2	49	110	8	118
6. Skeleton (Upper Extremities)		38	6	44	54	4	58	92	10	102
7. Legs		42	8	50	40	6	46	82	14	96
8. Toes		46	3	49	45	2	47	91	5	96
9. Wrists		38	11	49	38	4	42	76	15	91
10. Forearm		45	4	49	32	8	40	77	12	89
11. Ankles		35	8	43	34	7	41	69	15	84
12. Face		38	7	45	31	6	37	69	13	82
13. Skeleton (Lower Extremities)		28	3	31	43	4	47	71	7	78
14. Chest		43	....	43	31	4	35	74	4	78
15. Knees		30	6	36	20	7	27	50	13	63
16. Elbows		21	3	24	25	3	28	46	6	52
17. Shoulders		21	1	22	22	3	25	43	4	47
18. Skeleton (Head and Neck)		18	....	18	21	4	25	39	4	43
19. Scalp		13	....	13	19	1	20	32	1	33
20. Perineum and Genitalia		21	....	21	8	....	8	29	....	29
21. Nose		11	1	12	10	1	11	21	2	23
22. Hip		8	3	11	11	1	12	19	4	23
23. Thigh		14	1	15	5	1	6	19	2	21
24. Arms		12	1	13	7	....	7	19	1	20
25. Mouth		9	....	9	10	....	10	19	....	19
26. Phalangeal Joints (Upper Extremities)		10	2	12	5	2	7	15	4	19
27. Neck		9	....	9	4	....	4	13	....	13
28. Jaw		4	....	4	5	....	5	9	....	9
29. Ears		5	....	5	3	....	3	8	....	8
30. Phalangeal Joints (Lower Extremities)		5	1	6	1	....	1	6	1	7
31. Abdomen		4	....	4	1	1	2	5	1	6
32. Internal Injuries		5	....	5	1	....	1	6	1	7
33. Teeth		2	....	2	2	....	2	4	....	4
34. Skeleton (Trunk)		1	....	1	2	....	2	3	....	3
Total Anatomical Units Injured		1365	185	1550	1167	138	1305	2532	324	2856
Total No. of Patients		1111	150	1261	904	102	1006	2015	252	2267
Ratio of Anatomical Units to Number of Patients		1.23	1.23	1.23	1.29	1.35	1.30	1.26	1.28	1.26

*Arranged in the order of frequency of the total for all ages.

TABLE 3.2

PARTS OF BODY INJURED IN INDUSTRIAL ACCIDENTS IN 1947–1948

(*71*) (*National Safety Council*)

Parts of Body	Per cent of Cases	Per cent of Compensation
Eyes	5%	3%
Head	6%	9%
Arms	9%	11%
Trunk	24%	26%
Hands	8%	6%
Fingers	18%	14%
Legs	11%	13%
Teeth	9%	7%
Toes	5%	2%
General	5%	9%

TABLE 3.3

PARTS OF BODY INJURED IN NON-INDUSTRIAL ACCIDENTS BY AGE AND SEX*, 1946-48

Anatomical Units Injured	Under 35 M	Under 35 F	Under 35 T	35 and Older M	35 and Older F	35 and Older T	Total All Ages M	Total All Ages F	Total All Ages T
1. Fingers	174	99	273	79	32	111	253	131	384
2. Face	140	78	218	42	15	57	182	93	275
3. Eyes	117	59	176	57	29	86	174	88	262
4. Hands	118	37	155	47	19	66	165	56	221
5. Scalp	91	43	134	42	14	56	133	57	190
6. Skeleton (Upper Extremities)	59	18	77	31	20	51	90	38	128
7. Legs	34	41	75	16	18	34	50	59	109
8. Knees	42	27	69	16	22	38	58	49	107
9. Mouth	56	21	77	20	8	28	76	29	105
10. Forearm	49	30	79	17	6	23	66	36	102
11. Ankles	42	27	69	17	15	32	59	42	101
12. Feet	40	34	74	17	8	25	57	42	99
13. Chest	29	16	45	32	10	42	61	26	87
14. Wrist	28	20	48	7	11	18	35	31	66
15. Elbow	28	18	46	14	6	20	42	24	66
16. Arms	29	18	47	9	6	15	38	24	62
17. Shoulder	27	16	43	11	7	18	38	23	61
18. Back (Lumbar)	26	14	40	14	7	21	40	21	61
19. Nose	29	15	44	10	3	13	39	18	57
20. Toes	12	18	30	7	7	14	19	25	44
21. Ears	21	10	31	4	3	7	25	13	38
22. Skeleton (Lower Extremities)	11	7	18	10	9	19	21	16	37
23. Neck	14	8	22	4	3	7	18	11	29
24. Skeleton (Head and Neck)	9	3	12	9	3	12	18	6	24
25. Skeleton (Trunk)	9	3	12	9	3	12	18	6	24
26. Hip	8	4	12	5	6	11	13	10	23
27. Thighs	7	9	16	6	....	6	13	9	22
28. Abdomen	11	8	19	....	2	2	11	10	21
29. Jaw	5	7	12	3	3	6	8	10	18
30. Teeth	8	6	14	....	1	1	8	7	15
31. Perineum-Genitalia	5	3	8	6	....	6	11	3	14
32. Phalangeal Joints (Upper Extremities)	7	5	12	1	....	1	8	5	13
33. Phalangeal Joints (Lower Extremities)	....	....	....	3	2	5	3	2	5
34. Internal Injuries	2	1	3	....	2	2	2	3	5
Total Anatomical Units Injured	1287	723	2010	565	300	865	1852	1023	2875
Total No. of Patients	942	478	1420	400	193	593	1342	671	2013
Ratio of Anatomical Units to Number of Patients	1.37	1.51	1.41	1.41	1.55	1.46	1.38	1.52	1.43

*Arranged in the order of frequency of the total for all ages.

TABLE 3.4

Parts of Body Injured in Industrial and Non-Industrial Accidents by Age and Sex

Number of Anatomical Units

| Part of Body Injured | Industrial Accidents 1947 ||||||||| Non-Industrial Accidents 1946-48 |||||||||
| | Under 35 ||| 35 and Older ||| Total All Ages ||| Under 35 ||| 35 and Older ||| Total All Ages |||
Age / Sex	M	F	T	M	F	T	M	F	T	M	F	T	M	F	T	M	F	T
Upper Extremities	631	116	747	560	81	641	1191	197	1388	519	261	780	216	107	323	735	368	1103
Head and Neck	332	24	356	258	17	275	590	41	631	490	250	740	191	82	273	681	332	1013
Lower Extremities	271	39	310	246	30	276	517	69	586	196	167	363	97	87	184	293	254	547
Trunk	131	6	137	103	10	113	234	16	250	82	43	125	61	24	85	143	67	210
Total Parts of Body	1365	185	1550	1167	138	1305	2532	323	2855	1287	721	2008	565	300	865	1852	1021	2873
Total Number Patients	1111	150	1261	904	102	1006	2015	252	2267	942	478	1420	400	193	593	1392	671	2063

TABLE 4.1

COMMON TYPES OF NON-INDUSTRIAL ACCIDENTS BY AGE 1930–1948

Type or Manner	1 Falls	2 Aggressive Behavior	3 Handling Objects	4 Foreign Bodies in Orifices	5 Motor Vehicles	6 Bumping Into Objects	7 Dropping Objects	8 Animal Bites	Per Cent Total
Per cent of Total	21.2	17.0	12.0	11.6	8.9	7.1	5.7	4.2	87.7
Age									
0–4	37.6*	7.9	4.6	11.8†	5.0	10.2‡	8.0	4.3	89.4
5–9	27.7*	12.6†	7.3	6.7	9.6‡	8.4	5.2	9.1	86.6
10–14	31.1*	10.0	11.4‡	6.3	7.5	7.5	4.9	10.2‡	88.9
15–19	20.3*	16.8†	12.9‡	10.9	11.4	6.6	7.2	4.1	90.2
20–24	12.4‡	27.1*	13.8†	11.9	9.7	5.9	3.9	2.4	87.1
25–29	12.9†	22.6*	11.7	12.5‡	10.4	6.1	7.3	2.0	85.5
30–34	14.5†	22.9*	13.0‡	12.9†	7.6	6.4	6.0	2.5	85.8
35–39	14.5	18.9*	17.6†	15.7‡	7.8	7.3	4.0	3.2	89.0
40–44	20.0*	14.1	15.5†	14.6‡	9.3	8.1	6.2	2.4	90.2
45–49	22.3*	11.9	12.4‡	12.9†	8.4	6.3	6.6	4.2	85.0
50–54	23.8*	14.5†	11.6‡	11.7‡	8.1	8.1	5.3	2.8	85.9
55–59	24.4*	6.4	13.4‡	13.9†	9.9	4.7	7.0	5.8	85.5
60–64	29.8*	16.8†	12.2	11.5	13.0‡	6.1	0.8	2.3	92.5
65–69	40.3*	12.9†	9.6‡	9.8‡	8.1	3.2	4.8	4.8	93.5
70–74	39.2*	.....	7.8	2.0	9.8‡	11.8†	3.9	11.8†	86.3
75†	54.6*	3.0	3.0	......	15.2	3.0	3.0	15.2†	97.0

*Most frequent types of accidents for given age group.
†Second most frequent types of accidents for given age group.
‡Third most frequent types of accidents for given age group.

TABLE 4.2
Types of Non-Industrial Accidents, Groups A, B and A & B 1930 - 1948

Number of Cases

Manner of Accident	Group A 0-34 M	F	T	Group A 35† M	F	T	Group A Total M	F	T	Group B 0-34 M	F	T	Group B 35† M	F	T	Group B Total M	F	T	Groups A & B 0-34 M	F	T	Groups A & B 35† M	F	T
1. Fall on level	205	132	337	105	104	209	310	236	546	147	100	247	50	22	72	197	122	319	352	232	584	155	126	281
2. Fall from height	128	100	228	69	70	139	197	170	367	102	57	159	31	9	40	133	66	199	230	157	387	100	79	179
3. Dropped object	119	63	182	54	19	73	173	82	255	61	38	99	33	1	34	94	39	133	180	101	281	87	20	107
4. Bumped into object	135	76	211	82	34	116	217	110	327	78	43	121	22	9	31	100	52	152	213	119	332	104	43	147
5. Struck by moving vehicle	188	109	297	104	53	157	292	162	454	79	43	122	16	14	30	95	57	152	267	152	419	120	67	187
6. Stepped on object	56	32	88	18	12	30	74	44	118	53	22	75	5	2	7	58	24	82	109	54	163	23	14	37
7. Turned or twisted	51	29	80	50	29	79	101	58	159	31	24	55	14	5	19	45	29	74	82	53	135	64	34	98
8. Handling objects																								
a. household utensils	50	87	137	33	59	92	83	146	229	48	53	101	10	13	23	58	66	124	98	140	238	43	72	115
b. tools and machinery	92	11	103	75	7	82	167	18	185	55	4	59	28	1	29	83	5	88	147	15	162	103	8	111
c. other objects	47	14	61	47	5	52	94	19	113	37	18	55	16	3	19	53	21	74	84	32	116	63	8	71
9. Foreign body in body orifice																								
a. put into orifice	47	32	79	13	16	29	60	48	108	27	20	47	3	3	6	30	23	53	74	52	126	16	19	35
b. flew into orifice	197	91	288	153	55	208	350	146	496	64	23	87	27	10	37	91	33	124	261	114	375	180	65	245
10. Aggression																								
a. fights and attacks	249	71	320	135	31	166	384	102	486	270	108	378	92	22	114	362	130	492	519	179	698	227	53	280
b. miscellaneous aggression	82	22	104	5	6	11	87	28	115	31	5	36	3	2	5	34	7	41	113	27	140	8	8	16
c. parental aggression	4	9	13	…	…	…	4	9	13	3	4	7	…	…	…	3	4	7	7	13	20	…	…	…
11. Self-aggression																								
a. impulsive and violent	18	4	22	2	…	2	20	4	24	8	10	18	3	2	5	11	12	23	26	14	40	5	2	7
b. scratching, probing, rubbing	23	16	39	12	4	16	35	20	55	10	10	20	3	4	7	13	14	27	33	26	59	15	8	23
12. Animal bites, etc	67	46	113	45	16	61	112	62	174	66	30	96	7	5	12	73	35	108	133	76	209	52	21	73
13. Fingers caught in door	20	12	32	20	12	32	40	24	64	13	14	27	7	1	8	20	15	35	33	26	59	27	13	40
14. Miscellaneous	62	41	103	32	9	41	94	50	144	15	13	28	6	…	6	21	13	34	77	54	131	38	9	47
Total	1840	997	2837	1054	541	1595	2894	1538	4432	1198	639	1837	376	128	504	1574	767	2341	3038	1636	4674	1430	669	2099

Table 4.3

Principal Means of Industrial Accidents by Severity of Injury and Extent of Disability in 1947–1948

(71)   (National Safety Council)

Means of Accident in all Disabling Injuries		Temporary Total	Permanent Partial	Fatal *and* Permanent Total
Handling objects	22%	26%	10%	....
Falls	17%	18%	14%	19%
Machinery	16%	10%	32%	9%
Falling objects	13%	11%	18%	10%
Motor-vehicles	7%	....	7%	22%
Hand tools	7%	7%	8%	....
Striking against object	....	7%	....	....
Electricity, explosives, etc.	....	....	....	9%
Harmful substances	....	....	....	7%
Others	18%	21%	11%	24%
TOTAL	100%	100%	100%	100%

Table 4.4

Principal Means of Fatal Home Accidents in 1951

(71)   (National Safety Council)

Types	Total Deaths	Rate	Where Encountered
Falls	14,700	9.6	Affects mainly older age groups
Burns	5,000	3.3	Common at both extremes of life
Miscellaneous	3,700	2.4	
Mechanical suffocation	1,450	0.9	Ninety-five per cent under age of five; ninety per cent under age of one
Poisons	1,250	0.8	More than eighty per cent occur in the home
Poisonous gas	1,000	0.7	Affects mainly the aged and gas producing areas
Firearms	900	0.6	Forty per cent occur in the home

TABLE 4.5

CAUSES OF HOSPITALIZED HOME ACCIDENTS

(*51*) (*Rupp and Battey*)

Mechanical Causes	Personal Causes
1. Disorder.....................18%	1. Poor judgment..............24%
2. Improper equipment..........10%	2. Child injury, adult fault......10%
3. Improper use of equipment.....10%	3. Physical fraility.............. 8%
4. House needed repairs.......... 8%	4. Hurry...................... 6%
5. Ice on walk.................. 4%	5. Intoxication................. 5%
6. Lack of light................. 4%	6. Physical handicap........... 3%
7. Other mechanical............10%	7. Other personal..............12%
8. No mechanical factor..........36%	8. No personal cause...........32%

TABLE 5.1

INDUSTRIAL (1946–48) AND NON-INDUSTRIAL (1930–49) ACCIDENTS BY MONTH (MALE AND FEMALE)

Number of Accidents

Month \ Age	Industrial Accidents					Non-Industrial Accidents					
	15-29	30-44	45-59	60†	All Ages	0-14	15-29	30-44	45-59	60†	All Ages
January......	203	183	84	25	495	101	183	140	82	31	537
February	179	141	87	21	428	95	164	122	87	20	488
March.......	170	172	79	18	439	136	177	118	60	24	515
April........	217	173	97	25	512	191	231	178	75	25	700
May.........	203	179	74	28	484	192	185	147	63	29	616
June.........	217	187	108	33	545	251	317	178	91	25	862
July.........	253	210	97	14	574	272	306	194	84	21	877
August.......	263	212	106	24	605	269	297	204	100	37	907
September....	226	229	118	32	605	218	259	143	88	22	730
October......	230	208	97	24	559	163	246	182	98	27	716
November ...	239	199	93	25	556	143	235	167	73	29	647
December ...	222	192	100	18	532	97	238	168	75	35	613
TOTAL..	2622	2285	1140	287	6334	2128	2838	1941	976	325	8208

TABLE 5.2

Non-Industrial Accidents by Month, Age and Sex 1930–1948

Cases

Sex Month Age	Male 0–14	15–29	30–44	45–59	60+	All Ages	No Age	Total	Female 0–14	15–29	30–44	45–59	60+	All Ages	No Age	Total
January...	64	125	96	56	15	356	31	387	40	64	49	29	17	199	19	218
February.	52	97	74	50	9	282	38	320	38	58	41	32	10	179	15	194
March...	91	121	82	46	16	356	25	381	49	62	40	16	9	176	16	192
April.....	113	117	109	44	15	398	28	426	72	69	38	19	14	212	22	234
May......	137	165	121	49	12	484	37	521	60	74	63	28	14	239	15	254
June......	174	206	122	65	16	583	42	625	77	111	56	26	9	279	17	296
July......	192	193	147	60	11	603	37	640	89	123	53	27	11	303	23	326
August...	177	178	145	67	24	591	30	621	101	129	66	36	14	346	12	358
September	135	154	91	55	11	446	27	473	83	105	52	33	11	284	20	304
October..	107	170	140	63	12	492	31	523	61	84	48	38	16	247	11	258
November	89	151	116	56	24	436	25	461	54	84	51	17	5	211	22	233
December	66	159	116	53	24	418	26	444	34	87	57	24	12	214	16	230

TABLE 5.3

SEASONAL DISTRIBUTION OF INDUSTRIAL ACCIDENTS

(MALE AND FEMALE) 1946–1948

	Number					Percent				
Age	Winter	Spring	Summer	Autumn	Total	Winter	Spring	Summer	Autumn	Total
15–29	604	590	733	695	2622	23	23	28	26	100
30–44	516	524	609	636	2285	23	23	26	28	100
45–59	270	250	312	308	1140	24	22	27	27	100
60†	64	71	71	81	287	22	25	25	28	100
Total	1454	1435	1725	1720	6334	23	23	27	27	100

TABLE 5.4

SINGLE INDUSTRIAL ACCIDENTS BY MONTH AND AGE OF PATIENT (MALE) 1946–48

	Cases											
Month Age	Jan.	Feb.	Mar.	Apr.	May	June	July	Aug.	Sept.	Oct.	Nov.	Dec.
15–29	123	108	118	133	129	141	161	170	131	149	138	138
30–44	117	87	123	106	125	114	136	129	125	124	132	114
45–59	59	58	54	47	67	70	63	69	88	71	63	70
60†	18	17	13	20	21	26	10	20	18	19	19	14
TOTAL	317	270	308	306	342	351	370	388	362	363	352	336

TABLE 5.5

MULTIPLE INDUSTRIAL ACCIDENTS BY MONTH AND AGE OF PATIENT (MALE) 1946–48

	Cases											
Month Age	Jan.	Feb.	Mar.	Apr.	May	June	July	Aug.	Sept.	Oct.	Nov.	Dec.
15–29	48	42	42	59	45	57	69	68	64	51	51	40
30–44	52	31	37	53	38	55	56	72	76	62	43	54
45–59	18	19	13	21	20	21	23	31	15	16	20	22
60†	4	1	5	6	3	2	3	2	10	6	3	3
TOTAL	122	93	97	139	106	135	151	173	165	135	117	119

TABLE 5.6

SINGLE AND MULTIPLE INDUSTRIAL ACCIDENTS BY MONTH AND AGE OF PATIENT (FEMALE) 1946–48

| Month
Age | \multicolumn{12}{c}{Cases} ||||||||||||
	Jan.	Feb.	Mar.	Apr.	May	June	July	Aug.	Sept.	Oct.	Nov.	Dec.
15–29	32	19	16	25	29	19	23	34	23	38	42	44
30–44	14	15	18	14	16	18	18	18	20	29	17	24
45–59	7	5	14	6	10	17	11	10	11	13	7	8
60 †	3	2	.....	2	1	5	1	3	3	.....	2	1
TOTAL	56	41	48	47	56	59	53	65	57	80	68	77

TABLE 5.7

INCIDENCE OF ACCIDENTS BY MONTH IN 1948

(64) *(Wolff)*

Month	New Accidents	Man Hours Worked
January	1,036	600,160
February	954	552,495
March	1,272	646,201
April	1,095	558,854
May	1,140	580,803
June	1,311	567,802
July	1,527	607,594
August	1,602	629,156
September	1,343	644,743
October	1,338	720,941
November	1,266	690,720
December	941	565,987
TOTAL	14,825	7,365,456

Table 6.1

Half and Quarter Day Frequency of Industrial (1947) and Non-Industrial (1946–48) Accidents by Sex

Hours	Industrial M	Industrial F	Industrial T	Non-Industrial M	Non-Industrial F	Non-Industrial T	% Industrial M	% Industrial F	% Industrial T	% Non-Industrial M	% Non-Industrial F	% Non-Industrial T
am 6–12 n	787	111	898	144	74	218	42.2	46.2	42.7	16.7	18.0	17.1
n 12– 6 pm	899	111	1010	296	152	448	48.2	46.2	48.0	34.4	36.9	35.2
pm 6–12 mn	147	15	162	301	142	443	7.9	6.3	7.7	35.0	34.4	34.8
mn 12– 6 am	32	3	35	120	44	164	1.7	1.3	1.6	13.9	10.7	12.9
TOTAL	1865	240	2105	861	412	1273	100%	100%	100%	100%	100%	100%
am 6– 6 pm	1686	222	1908	440	226	666	90.4	92.5	90.6	51.1	54.9	52.3
pm 6– 6 am	179	18	197	421	186	607	9.6	7.5	9.4	48.9	45.1	47.7
TOTAL	1865	240	2105	861	412	1273	100%	100%	100%	100%	100%	100%

TABLE 6.2

Hour of Non-Industrial Accidents by Age and Sex 1930–48

Hour	0–19	20–34	35–49	50†
6 am	1	30	11	14
7	18	26	17	11
8	36	46	30	19
9	37	51	46	26
10	71	68	43	27
11	86	66	38	22
12 pm	89	72	40	23
1	105	59	48	19
2	109	72	43	24
3	130	88	65	30
4	118	68	53	20
5	126	95	61	26
6	121	82	34	23
7	103	77	52	19
8	109	107	66	17
9	90	116	34	22
10	45	118	50	17
11	31	108	42	18
12 am	18	69	33	10
1	22	60	18	9
2	18	70	27	9
3	4	44	15	5
4	4	20	13	2
5	4	13	2	6
TOTAL	1495	1625	881	418

TABLE 6.3

Hourly Per Cent Distribution of Total Accident Cases

(66) (Div. of Labor Statistics and Research of the State of California)

A.M. Hours	% Of All Injuries	P.M. Hours	% Of All Injuries
6–7	0.8	12–1	3.7
7–8	2.3	1–2	6.1
8–9	5.6	2–3	11.0
9–10	8.2	3–4	12.1
10–11	14.1	4–5	8.4
11–12	11.1	5–6	3.6

TABLE 6.4

HOUR OF INDUSTRIAL ACCIDENTS, 1947

	Cases			Per cent		
Hour	Male	Female	Total	Male	Female	Total
5 am	3	...	3	0.1	.....	0.1
6	9	...	9	0.5	.....	0.4
7	36	8	44	1.9	3.2	2.1
8	119	20	139	6.4	8.3	6.6
9	180	15	195	9.6	6.3	9.3
10	262	40	302	14.0	16.7	14.3
11	181	28	209	9.7	11.7	9.9
12 pm	85	15	100	4.6	6.2	4.7
1	159	19	178	8.5	7.9	8.5
2	195	23	218	10.5	9.6	10.4
3	243	23	266	13.0	9.6	12.6
4	148	24	172	7.9	10.0	8.2
5	69	7	76	3.7	2.9	3.6
6	25	4	29	1.3	1.7	1.4
7	20	1	21	1.1	0.4	1.0
8	36	3	39	1.9	1.3	1.9
9	16	1	17	0.9	0.4	0.8
10	24	4	28	1.3	1.7	1.3
11	26	2	28	1.4	0.9	1.4
12 am	7	1	8	0.4	0.4	0.4
1	3	...	3	0.2	.....	0.2
2	11	...	11	0.6	.....	0.5
3	5	...	5	0.3	.....	0.2
4	3	2	5	0.2	0.8	0.2
TOTAL	1865	240	2105	100%	100%	100%

TABLE 6.5

HOUR OF INDUSTRIAL ACCIDENTS BY AGE (MALE) 1948

Hour	15–19	20–24	25–29	30–34	35–39	40–44	45–49	50–54	55–59	60–64	65–69	70†	Total
6 am	...	...	...	2	...	...	2	1	..	..	..	..	5
7	2	3	3	5	3	2	5	2	..	3	1	..	29
8	3	22	18	15	9	8	11	2	2	2	..	1	93
9	16	20	30	28	16	19	9	16	12	4	4	3	177
10	19	40	45	35	30	31	21	16	6	10	3	..	256
11	13	26	18	32	26	17	14	5	10	4	..	1	166
12 n	6	17	17	11	8	9	5	6	1	1	..	..	81
1 pm	12	28	28	14	18	18	13	5	3	3	1	1	144
2	21	39	51	30	23	27	18	15	8	6	2	..	240
3	17	33	33	37	29	35	18	11	12	5	2	3	235
4	11	31	21	24	22	19	15	7	6	3	2	1	162
5	4	10	8	12	13	5	1	2	..	3	2	..	60
6	2	10	3	3	4	6	1	1	1	..	..	..	31
7	1	5	...	3	3	1	2	..	..	1	1	..	17
8	2	4	3	1	5	...	1	2	4	..	..	..	22
9	...	5	4	4	4	3	2	1	..	..	..	..	23
10	1	3	5	6	2	3	1	..	1	..	..	..	22
11	...	3	1	2	1	2	2	..	2	..	..	..	13
12 m	...	1	...	1	4	2	1	3	1	1	..	..	14
1 am	...	...	...	...	4	3	...	1	..	..	..	..	8
2	...	2	...	1	...	4	2	..	..	..	..	..	9
3	...	1	2	1	...	...	...	1	..	..	..	..	5
4	...	2	...	1	...	...	...	..	..	..	..	..	3
5	1	...	1	1	...	...	...	1	..	..	..	..	4
Total	131	305	291	269	224	214	144	98	69	46	18	10	1819

TABLE 6.6

HOUR OF INDUSTRIAL ACCIDENTS BY AGE (FEMALE) 1948

Hour	15–19	20–24	25–29	30–34	35–39	40–44	45–49	50–54	55–59	60–64	65–69	70†	Total
6 am	...	...	...	...	...	...	...	..	..	..	..	..	....
7	...	...	...	...	1	...	...	..	..	..	1	..	2
8	2	4	2	...	2	1	3	2	1	..	..	..	17
9	4	5	3	2	2	4	...	2	..	..	1	..	23
10	3	8	4	2	3	4	2	2	2	1	..	..	31
11	4	4	5	...	4	2	1	2	..	1	2	..	25
12 n	2	5	2	...	1	1	2	..	..	1	3	..	17
1 pm	4	5	...	...	1	1	2	..	..	..	..	..	13
2	3	6	7	2	4	1	2	1	1	..	..	..	27
3	7	1	1	...	1	4	2	1	2	..	..	..	19
4	2	1	1	...	...	2	...	1	..	1	..	..	8
5	...	1	1	...	...	...	...	..	..	..	..	..	2
6	...	1	1	...	...	...	1	1	..	..	..	..	4
7	...	...	...	...	...	...	...	..	..	..	..	..	....
8	1	...	...	...	1	...	...	..	..	..	..	..	2
9	1	...	...	...	...	...	...	..	..	..	..	..	1
10	...	1	...	...	...	...	...	..	..	..	..	..	1
11	...	1	1	...	...	...	...	..	..	1	..	..	3
12 m	...	2	...	...	...	...	...	..	..	..	..	..	2
1 am	...	...	...	...	...	...	...	..	..	..	..	..	....
2	...	...	...	...	...	...	...	..	..	..	..	..	....
3	...	...	...	...	...	...	...	..	..	..	..	..	....
4	...	...	...	...	...	...	...	..	..	..	..	..	....
5	...	...	...	...	...	1	...	..	..	..	..	..	1
Total	33	45	28	6	20	21	15	12	6	5	7	..	198

TABLE 6.7

HOUR OF SINGLE INDUSTRIAL ACCIDENTS BY AGE (MALES) 1948

Hour	15–19	20–24	25–29	30–34	35–39	40–44	45–49	50–54	55–59	60–64	65–69	70†	Total
6 am	...	...	...	2	...	...	2	1	..	..	..	..	5
7	2	3	2	2	2	2	5	2	..	3	1	..	24
8	2	11	14	9	6	4	8	2	2	2	..	1	61
9	13	13	24	15	10	14	9	12	11	3	3	2	129
10	17	32	32	20	20	22	18	15	5	8	3	..	192
11	9	21	14	23	18	12	11	4	8	3	..	..	123
12 n	6	12	13	9	7	8	4	5	1	1	..	..	66
1 pm	7	19	23	11	11	15	9	4	2	3	1	1	106
2	16	35	38	17	14	17	12	9	7	6	2	..	173
3	13	25	19	24	17	23	14	9	10	5	2	3	164
4	9	26	14	18	19	16	12	5	6	2	2	1	130
5	3	7	2	9	8	3	1	2	..	3	2	..	40
6	1	5	3	3	3	5	...	1	1	..	..	..	22
7	1	3	...	2	2	...	2	..	..	1	1	..	12
8	1	3	1	1	4	...	1	1	3	..	..	..	15
9	...	3	...	3	1	2	1	1	..	..	..	..	11
10	1	2	5	6	1	3	1	..	1	..	..	..	20
11	...	3	1	1	1	2	1	..	2	..	..	..	11
12 m	...	1	...	1	1	2	1	1	1	1	..	..	9
1 am	...	...	...	...	2	2	...	1	..	..	..	..	5
2	...	1	...	1	...	4	2	..	..	..	..	..	8
3	...	...	1	1	...	...	...	1	..	..	..	..	3
4	...	1	...	...	...	...	...	..	..	..	..	..	1
5	...	...	1	1	...	...	...	1	..	..	..	..	3
Total	101	226	207	179	147	156	114	77	60	41	17	8	1333

TABLE 6.8

HOUR OF SINGLE INDUSTRIAL ACCIDENTS BY AGE (FEMALE) 1948

	Age											
Hour	15–19	20–24	25–29	30–34	35–39	40–44	45–49	50–54	55–59	60–64	65–69	70†	Total
6 am	...	...	...	1	...	...	...	..	..	..	..	..	1
7	...	...	...	...	1	...	...	..	..	..	1	..	2
8	2	3	2	1	2	...	3	2	1	..	..	..	16
9	4	5	3	5	2	4	...	2	..	..	1	..	26
10	3	8	4	2	3	4	1	2	2	1	..	..	30
11	4	4	4	...	4	2	1	2	..	1	2	..	24
12 n	2	5	2	1	1	1	1	..	..	1	3	..	17
1 pm	4	5	...	2	1	1	2	..	..	..	..	..	15
2	3	6	7	7	4	1	2	1	1	..	..	..	32
3	7	1	1	2	1	4	2	1	2	..	..	..	21
4	2	1	1	...	...	2	...	1	..	1	..	..	8
5	...	1	1	...	...	...	...	..	..	..	..	..	2
6	...	1	1	...	...	...	1	1	..	..	..	..	4
7	...	...	...	...	...	...	...	..	..	..	..	..	...
8	1	...	...	...	1	...	...	..	..	..	..	..	2
9	1	...	...	...	...	...	...	..	..	..	..	..	1
10	...	1	...	...	...	...	...	..	..	..	..	..	1
11	...	1	1	...	...	...	...	..	..	1	..	..	3
12 m	...	2	...	...	...	...	...	..	..	..	..	..	2
1 am	...	...	...	...	...	...	...	..	..	..	..	..	...
2	...	...	...	...	...	...	...	..	..	..	..	..	...
3	...	...	...	...	...	...	...	..	..	..	..	..	...
4	...	...	...	...	...	...	...	..	..	..	..	..	...
5	...	...	...	...	...	1	...	..	..	..	..	..	1
Total	33	44	27	21	20	20	13	12	6	5	7	..	208

TABLE 6.9

HOUR OF MULTIPLE INDUSTRIAL ACCIDENTS BY AGE (MALE) 1948

Hour	15–19	20–24	25–29	30–34	35–39	40–44	45–49	50–54	55–59	60–64	65–69	70†	Total
6 am	...	...	...	...	...	...	...	..	..	..	..	..	...
7	...	...	1	3	1	...	...	..	..	..	..	..	5
8	1	11	4	6	3	4	3	..	..	..	..	..	32
9	3	7	6	13	6	5	...	4	1	1	1	1	48
10	2	8	13	15	10	9	3	1	1	2	..	..	64
11	4	5	4	9	8	5	3	1	2	1	..	1	43
12 n	...	5	4	2	1	1	1	1	..	..	..	..	15
1 pm	5	9	5	3	7	3	4	1	1	..	..	..	38
2	5	4	13	13	9	10	6	6	1	..	..	..	67
3	4	8	14	13	12	12	4	2	2	..	..	..	71
4	2	5	7	6	3	3	3	2	..	1	..	..	32
5	1	3	6	3	5	2	...	..	..	..	..	..	20
6	1	5	...	...	1	1	1	..	..	..	..	..	9
7	...	2	...	1	1	1	...	..	..	..	..	..	5
8	1	1	2	...	1	...	...	1	1	..	..	..	7
9	...	2	4	1	3	1	1	..	..	..	..	..	12
10	...	1	...	...	1	...	...	..	..	..	..	..	2
11	...	...	...	1	...	...	1	..	..	..	..	..	2
12 m	...	...	...	...	3	...	...	2	..	..	..	..	5
1 am	...	...	...	...	2	1	...	..	..	..	..	..	3
2	...	1	...	...	...	...	...	..	..	..	..	..	1
3	...	1	1	...	...	...	...	..	..	..	..	..	2
4	...	1	...	1	...	...	...	..	..	..	..	..	2
5	1	...	...	...	...	...	...	..	..	..	..	..	1
Total	30	79	84	90	77	58	30	21	9	5	1	2	486

TABLE 6.10

HOUR OF MULTIPLE INDUSTRIAL ACCIDENTS BY AGE (FEMALE) 1948

Hour	15–19	20–24	25–29	30–34	35–39	40–44	45–49	50–54	55–59	60–64	65–69	70†	Total
8 am	...	1	...	...	...	1	...	..	..	..	..	..	2
9	...	...	...	1	...	...	...	..	..	..	..	..	1
10	...	...	...	1	...	...	1	..	..	..	..	..	2
11	...	...	1	...	...	...	...	..	..	..	..	..	1
12 n	...	...	...	...	...	...	1	..	..	..	..	..	1
1 pm	...	...	...	...	...	...	...	..	..	..	..	..	....
2	...	...	...	1	...	...	...	..	..	..	..	..	1
Total	...	1	1	3	...	1	2	..	..	..	..	..	8

TABLE 6.11

HOUR OF MULTIPLE INDUSTRIAL AND NON-INDUSTRIAL ACCIDENTS, 1931-36

	\multicolumn{12}{c}{Cases}

	\multicolumn{6}{c}{Industrial Accidents}	\multicolumn{6}{c}{Non-Industrial Accidents}

	\multicolumn{3}{c}{Two Accidents Per Patient}	\multicolumn{3}{c}{Three or More Accidents Per Patient}	\multicolumn{3}{c}{Two Accidents Per Patient}	\multicolumn{3}{c}{Three or More Accidents Per Patient}

Hour of Accident	M	F	T	M	F	T	M	F	T	M	F	T
Identical*...	208	14	222	313	6	319	11	6	17	7	5	12
Nearly Identical**	102	6	108	60	2	62	27	17	44	9	1	10
Unidentical..	481	26	507	47	1	48	68	20	88	..	....	......
Total.....	791	46	837	420	9	429	106	43	149	16	6	22

*Identical—accidents occurring within one hour.
**Nearly identical—accidents occurring within two hours.

TABLE 6.12

SIX-HOURLY GROUPINGS OF SINGLE AND MULTIPLE NON-INDUSTRIAL ACCIDENTS BY SEX AND GROUPS A AND B, 1930–1948

	\multicolumn{8}{c}{Cases}

Group	\multicolumn{4}{c}{Group A}	\multicolumn{4}{c}{Group B}

Sex	\multicolumn{2}{c}{Male}	\multicolumn{2}{c}{Female}	\multicolumn{2}{c}{Male}	\multicolumn{2}{c}{Female}

Hour	Multiple	Single	Multiple	Single	Multiple	Single	Multiple	Single
6–11 am	52	353	25	190	27	137	8	51
12– 5 pm	102	613	49	321	65	275	29	129
6–11 pm	114	538	49	288	67	278	24	143
12– 5 am	26	189	9	69	15	130	10	47
Total	294	1693	132	868	174	820	71	370

TABLE 6.13

HOUR OF DAY AND SEASON OF YEAR OF NON-INDUSTRIAL ACCIDENTS 1930–48
(FIFTEEN YEARS OF AGE AND OLDER) BY SEX

Sex Month Hour	Male Dec. Feb.	Male Mar. May	Male June Aug.	Male Sept. Nov.	Female Dec. Feb.	Female Mar. May	Female June Aug.	Female Sept. Nov.	Male and Female Dec. Feb.	Male and Female Mar. May	Male and Female June Aug.	Male and Female Sept. Nov.	Total
6 am	6	11	9	9	8	1	4	5	14	12	13	14	53
7	15	11	3	6	13	5	12	2	28	16	15	8	67
8	14	16	22	14	17	13	12	8	31	29	34	22	116
9	20	22	35	27	10	11	6	15	30	33	41	42	146
10	21	27	35	28	6	10	14	11	27	37	49	39	152
11	21	15	28	26	12	10	17	21	33	25	45	47	150
12 pm	24	25	33	24	18	15	18	19	42	40	51	43	176
1	19	28	32	20	11	8	12	19	30	36	44	39	149
2	27	20	36	36	6	16	21	15	33	36	57	51	177
3	32	30	55	46	17	15	22	19	49	45	77	65	236
4	18	25	34	45	11	16	13	20	29	41	47	65	182
5	34	31	39	34	20	24	24	22	54	55	63	56	228
6	31	29	37	22	15	5	22	15	46	34	59	37	176
7	24	26	38	29	18	9	19	18	42	35	57	47	181
8	25	30	51	50	12	15	30	24	37	45	81	74	237
9	32	36	42	42	12	14	19	19	44	50	61	61	216
10	38	26	48	37	14	12	19	28	52	38	67	65	222
11	29	30	59	36	16	13	24	13	45	43	83	49	220
12 am	25	22	24	31	11	8	11	7	36	30	35	38	139
1	14	21	26	22	7	6	20	8	21	27	46	30	124
2	17	17	31	23	16	8	17	9	33	25	48	32	138
3	13	14	16	19	4	3	4	6	17	17	20	25	79
4	7	9	2	13	4	1	3	2	11	10	5	15	41
5	2	1	6	4	5	....	2	5	7	1	8	9	25
Total	508	522	741	643	283	238	365	330	791	760	1106	973	3630

Table 6.14

Industrial Accidents by Sex in Two-Hour Periods, 1947

	Cases			Per cent		
Hour	Male	Female	Total	Male	Female	Total
6– 7 am	45	8	53	2.4	3.3	2.5
8– 9	299	35	334	16.0	14.6	15.9
10–11	443	68	511	23.8	28.3	24.3
12– 1 pm	244	34	278	13.1	14.2	13.2
2– 3	438	46	484	23.5	19.2	23.0
4– 5	217	31	248	11.6	12.9	11.8
6– 7	45	5	50	2.4	2.1	2.4
8– 9	52	4	56	2.8	1.7	2.7
10–11	50	6	56	2.7	2.5	2.6
12– 1 am	10	1	11	0.5	0.4	0.5
2– 3	16	...	16	0.9	....	0.7
4– 5	6	2	8	0.3	0.8	0.4
Total	1865	240	2105	100%	100%	100%

Table 6.15

Two-Hour Periods of Non-Industrial Accidents by Sex, Groups A and B 1946–49

	Group A			Group B			Groups A & B					
Hour	M	F	T	M	F	T	M	F	T	M	F	T
5– 6 am	7	13	20	4	4	8	11	17	28			
7– 8	29	19	48	4	4	8	33	23	56			
9–10	70	31	101	26	8	34	96	39	135			
11–12	83	36	119	23	14	37	106	50	156	246	129	375
1 –2 pm	79	42	121	32	15	47	111	57	168			
3– 4	121	55	176	35	17	52	156	72	228			
5– 6	108	59	167	38	12	50	146	71	217			
7– 8	103	47	150	40	16	56	143	63	206	556	263	819
9–10	100	51	151	33	12	45	133	63	196			
11–12	80	15	95	33	7	40	113	22	135			
1– 2 am	57	18	75	21	13	34	78	31	109			
3– 4	31	6	37	12	2	14	43	8	51	367	124	491

TABLE 7.1

PERCENTAGE OF INDUSTRIAL AND NON-INDUSTRIAL ACCIDENT PATIENTS BY PLACE OF RESIDENCE 1947

Patients	Office Neighborhood	Periphery and Downtown	Suburbs and Greater Cincinnati	Rural Areas	Per cent
Group A	42.8	17.0	34.4	5.8	100%
Group B	62.8	21.8	13.7	1.7	100%
Industrial	12.6	23.7	59.2	4.5	100%

TABLE 7.2

INDUSTRIAL ACCIDENTS BY TYPES OF INDUSTRY AND SEX 1948

Industry	Number Patients	Per cent
1. Metal goods, tools and machinery	414	18.6
2. Leather, wood, paper and glass products	181	8.1
3. Foods and beverages	99	4.4
4. Needle Trades	98	4.4
5. Chemicals	35	1.6
Total Manufacturing	(827)	(37.1)
6. Autos and appliances	402	18.0
7. Retail and wholesale trade	294	13.2
8. Construction and wrecking	200	9.0
9. Personal Service (hotels, amusements, laundry, cleaning)	127	5.7
10. Printing, engraving and lithographing	121	5.4
11. Trucking, freight handling, etc.	96	4.3
12. Public utility and transportation	71	3.2
13. Restaurants and cafes	69	3.1
14. Building maintenance and miscellaneous	21	1.0
Total	2228	100%

TABLE 7.3

INDUSTRIAL ACCIDENTS BY NUMBER OF ACCIDENTS PER FIRM
AND NUMBER OF FIRMS, 1948

Number of Accidents Per Firm	Firm Number	Per cent	Accidents Number	Per cent
1	335	(54.6)	335	(15.3)
2	99		198	
3	52		156	
4	31		124	
5	22		110	
1–5	539	87.7	923	42.3
6–10	33	5.4	247	11.4
11–15	15	2.6	200	9.2
16–25	14	2.2	257	11.7
26–49	9	1.5	273	12.5
50 plus	4	0.6	283	12.9
Total	614	100%	2183	100%

TABLE 8.1

PERCENTAGE OF NON-INDUSTRIAL (GROUPS A & B) AND INDUSTRIAL INJURIES
IN RELATION TO CINCINNATI'S POPULATION (1946–1948)

Age	Cincinnati Population		%A		%B		%A&B		Industrial Injuries**	
0–4	6.2		9.1		8.3		8.9			
5–9	6.2		7.4		6.3		7.1		22.0*	
10–14	7.1		5.0		8.1		6.0			
15–19	7.7		6.9		12.5		8.6		6.4	
20–24	8.3		15.2		17.6		16.0		14.5	
25–29	8.6		14.5		12.5		13.9		12.6	
30–34	8.5	52.6	10.0	68.1	10.5	75.8	10.1	70.6	9.9	65.4
35–39	8.0		9.5		9.2		9.4		9.8	
40–44	7.7		5.0		5.4		5.1		7.3	
45–49	7.3		5.5		3.5		4.9		6.5	
50–54	6.4		3.5		2.7		3.3		4.7	
55–59	5.2		2.7		1.4		2.3		2.7	
60–64	4.3		2.7		1.0		2.1		2.0	
65–69			1.4		0.8		1.2		1.2	
70–74	8.5		1.1		0.0		0.7		.2	
75–79		47.4	0.5	31.9	0.2	24.2	0.4	29.4	.2	34.6
			100%		100%		100%		100%	

* % of A & B, ages 0–14.
**Percentages corrected for comparison with home injuries.

TABLE 9.1

SINGLE AND MULTIPLE INDUSTRIAL ACCIDENTS BY SEX IN SINGLE YEAR GROUPS, 1930-1948 SERIES

Year	Accidents M	Accidents F	Accidents M&F	Patients M	Patients F	Patients M&F	Single Accidents Per Patient M	Single Accidents Per Patient F	Single Accidents Per Patient M&F	Multiple Accidents M	Multiple Accidents F	Multiple Accidents M&F	Patients With Multiple Accidents M	Patients With Multiple Accidents F	Patients With Multiple Accidents M&F
1948	1937	247	2184	1613	238	1851	1358	229	1587	579	18	597	255	9	264
1947	2076	256	2332	1718	240	1958	1450	226	1676	626	30	656	268	14	282
1946	1552	215	1767	1328	203	1531	1160	193	1353	392	22	414	168	10	178
1945	1506	240	1746	1283	229	1512	1117	218	1335	389	22	411	166	11	177
1944	1747	282	2029	1421	254	1675	1190	233	1423	557	49	606	231	21	252
1943	1894	294	2188	1533	274	1807	1280	255	1535	614	39	653	253	19	272
1942	1836	177	2013	1531	169	1700	1311	161	1472	525	16	541	220	8	228
1941	1849	135	1984	1544	133	1677	1302	131	1433	547	4	551	242	2	244
1940	1173	95	1268	1018	93	1111	895	91	986	278	4	282	123	2	125
1939	1002	123	1125	893	117	1010	802	113	915	200	10	210	91	4	95
1938	1112	133	1245	973	129	1102	865	126	991	247	7	254	108	3	111
1937	1617	152	1769	1369	148	1517	1167	144	1311	450	8	458	202	4	206
1936	1543	175	1718	1334	167	1501	1167	159	1326	376	16	392	167	8	175
1935	894	137	1031	743	129	872	630	121	751	264	16	280	113	8	121
1934	707	88	795	627	86	713	554	84	638	153	4	157	73	2	75
1933	575	55	630	483	53	536	414	51	465	161	4	165	69	2	71
1932	539	30	569	440	25	465	363	21	384	176	9	185	77	4	81
1931	470	30	500	388	30	418	323	30	353	147	...	147	65	...	65
1930	435	39	474	364	37	401	309	35	344	126	4	130	55	2	57
Total	24464	2903	27367	20603	2754	23357	17657	2621	20278	6807	282	7089	2946	133	3079

TABLE 9.2

INDUSTRIAL PATIENTS WITH SINGLE AND MULTIPLE ACCIDENTS BY SEX (1930–1948)

Sex	Total Patients	Single Accidents	Multiple Accidents	Accidents Per Patient							
				2	3	4	5	6	7	10	4†
Male....	20603	17657	2946	2326	440	112	39	15	12	2	180
Female..	2754	2621	133	122	6	5	....	....	....	....	5
Total ...	23357	20278	3079	2448	446	117	39	15	12	2	185

Per cent

Male....	100.0	85.7	14.3	11.3	2.1	0.5	0.2	0.07	0.05	0.01	0.8
Female..	100.0	95.2	4.8	4.4	0.2	0.2	....	....	....	....	0.2
Per cent Increase, Male over Female		197.9		156.8	950.0	150.0	....	....	....	....	300.0

TABLE 9.3

NON-INDUSTRIAL PATIENTS WITH MULTIPLE ACCIDENTS IN GROUPS A AND B, 1930–1948

Group	Total Number of Patients			Single Accidents Per Patient			Total Number Patients With Multiple Accidents			2 Accidents Per Patient			3 Accidents Per Patient			4† Accidents Per Patient		
	M	F	M&F	M	F	M&F	M	F	M&F	M	F	M&F	M	F	M&F	M	F	M&F
A	3156	1690	4846	2931	1580	4511	225	110	335	193	96	289	26	9	35	6	5	11
B	1373	712	2085	1235	645	1880	138	67	205	103	44	147	20	14	34	15	9	24
Total......	4529	2402	6931	4166	2225	6391	363	177	540	296	140	436	46	23	69	21	14	35

Per cent

	M	F	M&F	M	F	M&F	M	F	M&F	M	F	M&F	M	F	M&F	M	F	M&F
A	100.0	100.0	100.0	92.9	93.5	93.1	7.1	6.5	6.9	6.1	5.7	6.0	0.8	0.5	0.7	0.2	0.3	0.2
B	100.0	100.0	100.0	89.9	90.6	90.2	10.1	9.4	9.8	7.5	6.2	7.1	1.5	2.0	1.6	1.1	1.3	1.2
Per cent of Increase of B over A.....							42.2	44.6	42.0	22.9	18.3	18.3	87.5	300.0	128.5	450.0	333.0	500.0
Per cent A and B.........				92.0	92.6	92.2	8.0	7.4	7.8	67.9	32.1	100.0						
Per cent M&F	65.3	34.7	100.0	65.2	34.8	100.0	67.2	32.8	100.0				66.7	33.3	100.0	60.0	40.0	100.0

139

TABLE 9.4

CUMULATIVE PERCENTAGE OF INDUSTRIAL SINGLE AND MULTIPLE ACCIDENTS BY SEX AND AGE, 1930-1948

Age Group	Single										Multiple									
	Male			Female			Male and Female			Male			Female			Male and Female		
		Per cent			Per cent			Per cent			Per cent			Per cent			Per cent	
	No. Pts.	Total	Cumul.	No. Pts.	Total	Cumul.	No. Pts.	Total	Cumul.	No. Pts.	Total	Cumul.	No. Pts.	Total	Cumul.	No. Pts.	Total	Cumul.
15-19	1562	8.8	8.8	463	17.7	17.7	2025	10.0	10.0	34	6.5	6.5	24	18.0	18.0	58	8.8	8.8
20-24	2734	15.5	24.3	561	21.4	39.1	3295	16.2	26.2	90	17.2	23.7	36	27.1	45.1	126	19.2	28.0
25-29	2902	16.4	40.7	406	15.5	54.6	3308	16.3	42.5	91	17.4	41.1	27	20.3	65.4	118	18.0	46.0
30-34	2596	14.7	55.4	287	10.9	65.5	2883	14.2	56.7	85	16.3	57.4	8	6.0	71.4	93	14.2	60.2
35-39	2258	12.8	68.2	277	10.6	76.1	2535	12.5	69.2	69	13.2	70.6	9	6.8	78.2	78	11.9	72.1
40-44	1785	10.1	78.3	204	7.8	83.9	1989	9.8	79.0	59	11.3	81.9	13	9.8	88.0	72	11.0	83.1
45-49	1333	7.5	85.8	141	5.4	89.3	1474	7.3	86.3	39	7.5	89.4	8	6.0	94.0	47	7.2	90.3
50-54	1003	5.7	91.5	139	5.3	94.6	1142	5.6	91.9	30	5.7	95.1	3	2.2	96.2	33	5.0	95.3
55-59	726	4.1	95.6	77	2.9	97.5	803	4.0	95.9	13	2.5	97.6	3	2.2	98.4	16	2.4	97.7
60-64	447	2.5	98.1	34	1.3	98.8	481	2.4	98.3	7	1.3	98.9	1	0.8	99.2	8	1.2	98.9
65-69	207	1.2	99.3	24	0.9	99.7	231	1.1	99.4	5	0.9	99.8	1	0.8	100.0	6	0.9	99.8
70-74	82	0.5	99.8	6	0.2	99.9	88	0.4	99.8	1	0.2	100.0			100.0	1	0.2	100.0
75†	22	0.1	99.9	2	0.1	100.0	24	0.1	99.9			100.0			100.0			100.0
0-75†	17657	99.9		2621	100.0		20278	99.9		523	100.0		133	100.0		656	100.0	

140

TABLE 9.5

SINGLE AND MULTIPLE INDUSTRIAL ACCIDENTS BY AGE, YEAR AND SEX (1946-48)

Age	MALE 1948 Mult.	MALE 1948 Sing.	MALE 1948 Total	MALE 1947 Mult.	MALE 1947 Sing.	MALE 1947 Total	MALE 1946 Mult.	MALE 1946 Sing.	MALE 1946 Total	MALE 1946 Cor.*	MALE 1946-48 Mult.	MALE 1946-48 Sing.	MALE 1946-48 Total	MALE 1946-48 Cor.*	FEMALE 1948 Mult.	FEMALE 1948 Sing.	FEMALE 1948 Total	FEMALE 1947 Mult.	FEMALE 1947 Sing.	FEMALE 1947 Total	FEMALE 1946 Mult.	FEMALE 1946 Sing.	FEMALE 1946 Total	FEMALE 1946-48 Mult.	FEMALE 1946-48 Sing.	FEMALE 1946-48 Total
15-19	36	103	139	54	96	150	24	64	88	109	114	263	377	398	. .	34	34	6	35	41	4	32	36	10	101	111
20-24	97	232	329	106	272	378	68	170	238	281	271	674	945	988	6	44	50	2	55	57	. .	42	42	8	141	149
25-29	93	219	312	110	247	357	65	215	280	. .	268	681	949	. .	4	29	33	4	23	27	2	23	25	10	75	85
30-34	99	176	275	98	179	277	61	174	235	. .	258	529	787	. .	4	27	31	2	20	22	. .	19	19	6	66	72
35-39	82	157	239	68	193	261	53	126	179	. .	203	476	679	. .	. .	25	25	4	23	27	. .	24	24	4	72	76
40-44	68	162	230	71	127	198	35	128	163	. .	174	417	591	. .	. .	23	23	10	22	32	6	17	23	16	62	78
45-49	36	116	152	53	117	170	36	99	135	. .	125	332	457	. .	2	14	16	2	17	19	4	11	15	8	42	50
50-54	27	81	108	34	95	129	9	82	91	. .	70	258	328	. .	. .	13	13	. .	16	16	5	10	15	5	39	44
55-59	10	65	75	15	60	75	19	59	78	. .	44	184	228	. .	. .	8	8	8	8	16	. .	8	8	. .	24	24
60-64	6	41	47	8	48	56	20	29	49	. .	34	118	152	. .	. .	5	5	4	4	8	. .	5	5	. .	14	14
65-69	2	17	19	7	23	30	2	19	21	. .	11	59	70	. .	. .	4	4	3	3	. .	. .	. .	. .	7	7
70-74	2	9	11	. .	7	7	. .	10	10	. .	2	26	28	. .	. .	1	1	. .	. .	. .	1	1	. .	2	2
75†	. .	3	3	. .	5	5	. .	2	2	. .	. .	10	10	. .	. .	1	1	. .	. .	. .	. .	. .	. .	1	1
15-34	325	730	1055	368	794	1162	218	623	841	905	911	2147	3058	3122	14	134	148	14	133	147	6	116	122	34	383	417
35†	233	651	884	256	675	931	174	554	728	728	663	1880	2543	2543	2	94	96	16	93	109	15	76	91	33	263	296
15-75†	558	1381	1939	624	1469	2093	392	1177	1569	1633	1574	4027	5601	5665	16	228	244	30	226	256	21	192	213	67	646	713

*See Note Table 1.1.

141

Table 9.6

Industrial Patients by Sex, Age and Number of Accidents, 1948

Number of Patients With

Age	1 Accident M	1 Accident F	M&F	2 Accidents M	2 Accidents F	M&F	3 Acdts M	4 Acdts M	5 Acdts M	6 Acdts M	7 Acdts M
15–19	103	35	138	11	.	11	2	1	...	...	...
20–24	233	43	276	42	3	45	3	1	...	...	...
25–29	210	30	240	36	2	38	6	1	...	...	1
30–34	167	27	194	31	2	33	9	2	...	2	...
35–39	151	25	176	28	...	28	8	2	...	...	...
40–44	160	21	181	23	1	24	2	2	...	1	...
45–49	117	14	131	13	1	14	2	...	...	...	...
50–54	84	14	98	14	...	14	1	...	...	...	...
55–59	65	8	73	4	...	4	1	...	...	...	...
60–64	41	5	46	3	...	3	..	...	...	...	...
65–69	15	5	20	2	...	2	..	...	...	...	...
70–74	9	1	10	1	...	1	..	...	...	...	...
75†	3	1	4	...	...	...	..	...	...	...	...
Total	1358	229	1587	208	9	217	34	9	...	3	1

TABLE 9.7

PERCENTAGE OF SINGLE AND MULTIPLE INDUSTRIAL ACCIDENTS BY AGE AND YEAR (MALE) 1946, 1947, 1948

Age	1948 % Mult.	1948 % Sing.	1948 % Total	1948 Cum. Mult.	1948 Cum. Sing.	1948 Cum. Total	1947 % Mult.	1947 % Sing.	1947 % Total	1947 Cum. Mult.	1947 Cum. Sing.	1947 Cum. Total	1946 % Mult.	1946 % Sing.	1946 % Total	1946 Cum. Mult.	1946 Cum. Sing.	1946 Cum. Total
15–19	6.5	7.5	7.2	6.5	7.5	7.2	8.7	6.5	7.2	8.7	6.5	7.2	6.1	5.4	5.6	6.1	5.4	5.6
20–24	17.4	16.8	17.0	23.9	24.3	24.2	17.0	18.5	18.1	25.7	25.0	25.3	17.3	14.4	15.2	23.4	19.8	20.8
25–29	16.7	15.9	16.1	40.6	40.2	40.3	17.6	16.8	17.1	43.3	41.8	42.4	16.6	18.3	17.8	40.0	38.1	38.6
30–34	17.7	12.7	14.2	58.3	52.9	54.4	15.7	12.2	13.2	59.0	54.0	55.6	15.6	14.8	15.0	55.6	52.9	53.6
35–39	14.7	11.4	12.3	73.0	64.3	66.7	10.9	13.1	12.5	69.9	67.1	68.1	13.5	10.7	11.6	69.1	63.6	65.2
40–44	12.2	11.7	11.9	85.2	76.0	78.6	11.4	8.6	9.5	81.3	75.7	77.6	8.9	10.8	10.4	78.0	74.4	75.6
45–49	6.5	8.4	7.8	91.7	84.4	86.4	8.5	8.0	8.1	89.8	83.7	85.7	9.2	8.4	8.6	87.2	82.8	84.2
50–54	4.8	5.9	5.6	96.5	90.3	92.0	5.4	6.5	6.2	95.2	90.2	91.9	2.3	7.0	5.8	89.5	89.8	90.0
55–59	1.8	4.7	3.9	98.3	95.0	95.9	2.4	4.1	3.6	97.6	94.3	95.5	4.8	5.0	5.0	94.3	94.8	95.0
60–64	1.1	3.0	2.4	99.4	98.0	98.3	1.3	3.3	2.7	98.9	97.6	98.2	5.1	2.5	3.1	99.4	97.3	98.1
65–69	0.4	1.2	1.0	99.8	99.2	99.3	1.1	1.6	1.4	100.0	99.2	99.6	0.5	1.6	1.3	99.9	98.9	99.4
70–74	0.3	0.7	0.6	100.1	99.9	99.9	....	0.5	0.3	....	99.7	99.9	....	0.8	0.6	....	99.7	100.0
75†	....	0.1	0.1	....	100.0	100.0	....	0.3	0.2	....	100.0	100.1	....	0.2	0.1	....	99.9	100.1

TABLE 9.8

RATIO OF NUMBER OF ACCIDENTS TO NUMBER OF PATIENTS BY YEAR AND SEX
(INDUSTRIAL CASES) 1930–1948

Year	Total Accidents Male	Female	Multiple Accidents Male	Female
1948	120	104	227	200
1947	121	106	234	214
1946	117	106	233	220
1945	117	105	234	200
1944	123	111	241	233
1943	124	107	243	205
1942	120	106	236	200
1941	120	102	226	200
1940	115	102	226	200
1939	112	105	220	250
1938	114	103	229	230
1937	118	103	223	200
1936	116	105	225	200
1935	120	106	234	200
1934	113	101	210	200
1933	119	104	233	200
1932	123	120	229	225
1931	121	100	226	...
1930	120	105	229	200
1930–1948	119	105	230	212

TABLE 9.9

NON-INDUSTRIAL PATIENTS BY NUMBER OF INJURIES, SEX AND AGE
(GROUPS A AND B) 1946–48

	Age 0–34								
	Group A			Group B			Groups A & B		
	M	F	M&F	M	F	M&F	M	F	M&F
Number Injured	617	325	942	325	153	478	942	478	1420
Number Injuries	880	435	1315	492	235	727	1372	670	2042
Ratio..........	143	134	140	151	154	152	146	140	144

	Age 35†								
	Group A			Group B			Groups A & B		
	M	F	M&F	M	F	M&F	M	F	M&F
Number Injured	282	159	441	118	34	152	400	193	593
Number Injuries	383	218	601	186	85	271	569	303	872
Ratio..........	136	137	136	158	250	178	142	157	147

	All Ages								
	Group A			Group B			Groups A & B		
	M	F	M&F	M	F	M&F	M	F	M&F
Number Injured	899	484	1383	443	187	630	1342	671	2013
Number Injuries	1263	653	1916	678	320	998	1941	973	2914
Ratio..........	140	135	139	153	171	158	145	145	145

Table 9.10

Industrial Patients by Number of Injuries, Sex and Age 1948

	Ages 0–34			Ages 35†			All Ages		
	M	F	M&F	M	F	M&F	M	F	M&F
Number Injured	1111	150	1261	904	102	1006	2015	252	2267
Number Injuries	1390	168	1558	1155	125	1280	2545	293	2838
Ratio	125	112	123	127	123	127	126	116	125

Table 9.11

Industrial Patients Having Single or Multiple Accidents in Two or More Consecutive Years, 1936 – 1941

	Number	Per cent
(Multiple accidents in one year only)	(491)	(46.7)
Patients with single or multiple accidents in 2 consecutive years	455	43.3
Patients with single or multiple accidents in 3 consecutive years	75	7.1
Patients with single or multiple accidents in 4 consecutive years	22	2.1
Patients with single or multiple accidents in 5 consecutive years	7	0.7
Patients with single or multiple accidents in 6 consecutive years	1	0.1
Total	1051	100.0

Table 9.12

Industrial Patients Having Single or Multiple Accidents in Any Two or More Years in a Six-Year Period (1936–1941)

	Number	Per cent
(Multiple accidents in one year only)	(491)	(36.7)
Patients with single or multiple accidents in any 2 years	643	48.0
Patients with single or multiple accidents in any 3 years	143	10.7
Patients with single or multiple accidents in any 4 years	41	3.0
Patients with single or multiple accidents in any 5 years	20	1.5
Patients with single or multiple accidents in any 6 years	1	0.1
Total	1339	100.0

TABLE 9.13

FREQUENCY OF RECURRENCE OF MULTIPLE ACCIDENTS IN THE SAME INDUSTRIAL PATIENTS IN THREE-YEAR PERIODS 1935–37, 1942–44 AND 1946–48

Accidents Recurring In

Year	Number of Patients With Multiple Accidents	Any 2 of 3 Consecutive Years			2 Consecutive Years		
		Years Compared With	Number of Patients Recurring	Per cent Recurring	Year Compared With	Number of Patients Recurring	Per cent Recurring
1946............	168	1947 and 1948	20	11.9	1947	16	9.5
1947............	268	1946 and 1948	44	16.4	1948	31	11.6
1948............	255	1946 and 1947	37	14.5			
1946–1948.......	691	Average					10.6
1942............	220	1943 and 1944	21	9.5	1943	19	8.6
1943............	253	1942 and 1944	43	17.0	1944	27	10.7
1944............	231	1942 and 1943	29	12.6			
1942–1944.......	704	Average					9.7
1935............	113	1936 and 1937	18	15.9	1936	12	10.6
1936............	167	1935 and 1937	22	13.2	1937	13	7.8
1937............	202	1936 and 1935	19	9.4			
1935–1937.......	482	Average					9.2

147

Table 9.14

Multiple Non-Industrial Accidents by Age and Sex and Groups A and B

	Cases								
	Group A			Group B			Groups A & B		
Age	M	F	M&F	M	F	M&F	M	F	M&F
0–4	57	45	102	48	20	68	105	65	170
5–9	81	27	108	101	43	144	182	70	252
10–14	73	37	110	85	36	121	158	73	231
15–19	67	27	94	47	42	89	114	69	183
20–24	85	27	112	44	49	93	129	76	205
25–29	53	35	88	44	13	57	97	48	145
30–34	63	32	95	36	6	42	99	38	137
35–39	77	34	111	26	8	34	103	42	145
40–44	60	36	96	5	8	13	65	44	109
45–49	74	31	105	14	3	17	88	34	122
50–54	52	16	68	8	4	12	60	20	80
55–59	30	12	42	10	8	18	40	20	60
60–64	9	10	19	8	2	10	17	12	29
65–69	12	1	13	...	2	2	12	3	15
70–74	4	4	8	...	...	...	4	4	8
75†	6	6	12	...	...	...	6	6	12
Total	803	380	1183	476	244	720	1279	624	1903

TABLE 9.15

Non-Industrial Patients by Age, Sex and Number of Accidents in Groups A and B, (1946 – 48)

	Group A — Number of Patients With											Group B — Number of Patients With												
	1 Acdt		2 Acdts		3 Acdts		4 Acdts		6 Acdts	1 Acdts		2 Acdts		3 Acdts		4 Acdts		5 Acdts		6 Acdts	
Age	M	F	M	F	M	F	M	F	M	M	F	M	F	M	F	M	F	M	F	M	F
0–4	87	82	11	11	1	..	..	..	..	41	29	5	..	1	5	..	..	..	..	..	..
5–9	64	48	12	22	1	..	..	..	..	36	22	6	3	2	9	..	..	1	1	..	2
10–14	53	30	4	15	2	..	..	..	..	35	18	6	2	1	8	..	1	..	..	..	..
15–19	79	49	3	10	..	2	..	..	..	45	33	6	4	..	10	1	1	..	..	..	..
20–24	178	92	10	4	1	1	..	1	..	92	45	7	3	2	10	1	1	1	..	..	..
25–29	162	95	8	13	1	1	..	..	..	52	39	8	1	..	9	3	..	..	..	..	..
30–34	109	58	4	11	2	1	..	1	1	53	21	4	..	2	4	1	..	..	..	..	..
35–39	115	55	12	10	..	1	1	..	..	48	16	2	1	..	3	2	..	..	..	..	..
40–44	58	40	3	12	1	..	..	1	..	29	11	1	1	..	1	..	..	..	..	..	..
45–49	47	40	8	6	1	..	..	..	..	21	7	1	1	..	2	..	..	..	..	..	..
50–54	41	25	5	10	1	1	..	..	..	20	2	1	..	2	..	1	..	..	..	..	..
55–59	26	21	1	5	..	..	..	..	..	5	4	..	2	..	3	1	..	..	..	..	..
60–64	31	14	..	3	..	..	..	..	..	6	1	1	1	..	2	..	..	..	..	..	..
65–69	12	13	..	..	..	..	..	..	..	2	..	..	..	..	..	..	..	..	..	..	..
70–74	9	12	1	2	1	..	..	..	..	1	..	..	..	..	1	..	..	..	..	..	..
75†	10	6	..	..	..	..	..	..	..	..	1	..	..	..	1	..	..	..	..	..	..
Total	1081	680	82	123	12	9	3	1	3	486	250	48	18	13	66	5	18	2	2	1	2	1	3

149

TABLE 9.16

FREQUENCY DISTRIBUTION OF SIX HUNDRED FORTY-SEVEN INDUSTRIAL ACCIDENTS ACCORDING TO NUMBER OF ACCIDENTS PER PATIENT COMPARED WITH THREE THEORETICAL POSSIBILITIES

(29) (*Greenwood and Woods*)

Number of Accidents	Observed Frequencies	Poisson Distribution	Negative Binomial	Neyman's Series
0	447	406	442	448
1	132	189	140	128
2	42	45	45	49
3	21	7	14	16
4	3	1	5	5
5	2	0.1	2	1
Total	647	648.1	648	647

TABLE 9.17

OBSERVED AND THEORETICAL DISTRIBUTION OF ACCIDENTS

(30) (*Greenwood and Yule*)

Number of Accidents Incurred	Number of Women Incurring Accidents	Accident Frequency when Distribution was		
		by Chance	Biased	of Unequal Liabilities
0	448	406	452	442
1	132	189	117	140
2	42	45	56	45
3	21 ⎫	7 ⎫	18 ⎫	14 ⎫
4	3 ⎬ 26	1 ⎬ 8.1	4 ⎬ 23	5 ⎬ 21
5	2 ⎭	0.1 ⎭	1 ⎭	2 ⎭
Total	648	648.1	648	648

"It will be seen that while two-thirds of the women concerned suffered no accidents at all, about a fifth suffered one accident, and a fifteenth suffered two accidents. The more frequent accidents, three to five in number, were suffered by twenty-six women, while on a purely chance distribution it was calculated that only eight of them should have suffered these multiple accidents. On the biased distribution and unequal liabilities distribution, however, the calculated frequency corresponds much more closely with actual observation; but an extension of the method of analysis to a number of other groups of workers showed that, on the whole, the unequal liabilities distribution gave the best agreement. For this and other reasons there can be no doubt that the munition women did not start equal, but that a few of them were, from the outset, distinctly accident-prone." (60)

TABLE 9.18

MEAN ACCIDENT FREQUENCY OF A GROUP OF SHUNTERS DURING THREE ONE-YEAR PERIODS OF OBSERVATION, AND THE EFFECT OF REMOVING WORKERS WITH THE HIGHEST ACCIDENT FREQUENCY RATES ON THE REMAINDER OF THE GROUP

(2) (Adelstein) and (7) (Arbous and Kerrich)

	1st Year	2nd Year	3rd Year
Mean accident rate for 104 men	0.557	0.355	0.317
After removing 10 men with highest rate in first year, i.e., 94 remaining men	0.393	0.361	0.329

TABLE 9.19

CORRELATION BETWEEN ACCIDENTS (MAJOR AND MINOR) IN TWO CONSECUTIVE PERIODS

(21) (Farmer and Chambers)

Correlation Between Accidents in Years	Omnibus and Trolley Bus Drivers			
	Group A	Group B	Group C	Group D
1 and 2	0.298	0.182	0.235	0.071
1 and 3	0.235	.....	0.063	0.058
1 and 4	0.177	.....	0.281	0.127
1 and 5	0.274	.....	.....	.....
2 and 3	0.328	.....	0.078	0.225
2 and 4	0.176	.....	0.195	0.251
2 and 5	0.265	.....	.....	.....
3 and 4	0.212	.....	0.016	0.296
3 and 5	0.273	.....	.....	.....
4 and 5	0.224	.....	.....	.....

TABLE 10.1

ILLNESS FROM ALL CAUSES, BY AGE AND SEX, AND GROUPS A AND B (1947 — 48)

| Group | Number of Cases |||||||||
| Group | Group A ||| Group B ||| Groups A&B |||
Age	M	F	M&F	M	F	M&F	M	F	M&F
0–4	136	162	298	46	40	86	182	202	384
5–9	61	55	116	14	17	31	75	72	147
10–14	45	27	72	13	21	34	58	48	106
15–19	77	118	195	41	47	88	118	165	283
20–24	217	206	423	80	83	163	297	289	586
25–29	154	112	266	34	46	80	188	158	346
30–34	106	105	211	46	30	76	152	135	287
35–39	96	107	203	15	19	34	111	126	237
40–44	107	49	156	14	16	30	121	65	186
45–49	78	39	117	10	7	17	88	46	134
50–54	68	25	93	9	8	17	77	33	110
55–59	39	27	66	8	9	17	47	36	83
60–64	27	15	42	4	3	7	31	18	49
65–69	17	21	38	4	1	5	21	22	43
70–74	8	9	17	1	...	1	9	9	18
75–79	7	5	12	...	...	...	7	5	12
80 †	3	4	7	...	...	...	3	4	7
Total	1246	1086	2332	339	347	686	1585	1433	3018

TABLE 11.1

COMPARISON OF PERCENTAGE OF PATIENTS HAVING MULTIPLE ACCIDENTS BETWEEN GROUP A AND GROUP B

Group	Total	Multiple	Percentage	Standard Error
A	4846	335	6.9	$\pm \sqrt{.13} = \pm .36$
B	2085	205	9.8	$\pm \sqrt{.42} = \pm .65$

Differences = 9.8 — 6.9 = 2.9

Standard Error of difference = $\pm \sqrt{(.36)^2 + (.65)^2} = \pm \sqrt{.55} = \pm .74$

Critical Ratio = $\dfrac{2.9}{.74}$ = 3.92

The Conclusion: Group A had significantly fewer patients having multiple accidents than Group B.

TABLE 11.2

COMPARISON OF AGE DISTRIBUTION OF NON-INDUSTRIAL ACCIDENT POPULATION 1930–1948 WITH CINCINNATI CENSUS OF 1940

Age	Census Population	Accident Population Observed (O)	Accident Population Expected (E)	(O-E)	(O-E)²	(O-E)²/E
0–4...........	28280	682	491	191	36481	74.30
5–9...........	28232	679	490	189	35721	72.90
10–14..........	32375	577	562	15	225	.40
15–19..........	35233	754	611	143	20449	33.47
20–24..........	37655	1175	653	522	272484	417.28
25–29..........	39204	967	680	287	82369	121.13
30–34..........	38655	716	670	46	2116	3.16
35–39..........	36440	682	632	50	2500	39.56
40–44..........	34818	472	604	−132	17424	28.85
45–49..........	33135	416	575	−159	25281	43.97
50–54..........	29265	283	508	−225	50625	99.66
55–59..........	23774	196	412	−216	46656	113.24
60–64..........	19924	145	346	−201	40401	116.77
65–69..........	15966	74	277	−203	41209	148.77
70–74..........	12222	58	212	−154	23716	111.87
75†............	11432	45	198	−153	23409	118.23
	456610	7921	7921			1543.56

$$X^2 = \sum \frac{(O-E)^2}{E}$$

For fifteen degrees of freedom at the 1% level of significance the X^2 value is 30.578. Since the X^2 value obtained is much greater than 30.578, it is concluded that, if the accident population did not differ from the industrial population, a random sample of 7921 could have been secured less than once in one hundred replicate random samples of size 7921.

Table 11.3

Correlation Between Hour of Occurrence of Industrial and Non-Industrial Injuries

Hour	Industrial	Non-Industrial	R^1*	R^2**	D***	D^2
6 pm	114	260	1	3	2	4
7	86	251	4	4	0	0
8	106	299	2	1	1	1
9	74	262	6	2	4	16
10	90	230	3	5	2	4
11	77	199	5	6	1	1
12	29	130	7	7	0	0
1 am	23	109	9	9	0	0
2	22	124	10	8	2	4
3	10	68	13	10	3	9
4	11	39	11.5	12	.5	.25
5	11	35	11.5	13	1.5	2.25
6	26	59	8	11	3	9
						50.50
						ΣD^2

* R^1 is rank order of industrial frequency.
** R^2 is rank order of non-industrial frequency.
*** D is absolute difference between R^1 and R^2.

$$\varrho = 1 - \frac{6\Sigma D^2}{N(N^2-1)}$$

$$= 1 - \frac{303}{13(168)}$$

$$= 1 - \frac{303}{2184} = 1 - .139$$

$$= .861 \ (r = .871)$$
(at 1% level, d.f. = 11, r = .684)
very significant*

* There is less than one chance in a hundred that no correlation exists between these two groups as to hourly distribution of injuries over the thirteen-hour period extending from 6 pm to 7 am.

TABLE 11.4

CORRELATION BETWEEN AGE DISTRIBUTIONS OF SELECTED SAMPLES

1. r* = .94 between 1930 and 1948 industrial accidents
2. r = .98 between 1946 and 1948 industrial accidents
3. r = .98 between 1940 and 1947–1948 industrial accidents
4. r = .98 between 1940 and 1930–1948 industrial accidents
5. r = .97 between industrial and non-industrial accidents, 1930–1948 samples
6. r = .91 between Groups A & B, non-industrial accidents, 1930–1948 samples
7. r = .92 between Groups A & B single accidents, 1930–1948 samples
8. r = .56 between Groups A & B multiple accidents, 1930–1948 samples
9. r = .96 between male and female non-industrial accidents of Group A, 1930–1948 samples
10. r = .94 between male and female non-industrial accidents of Group B, 1930–1948 samples
11. r = .97 between multiple non-industrial accidents of Group A, 1930–1948 samples, as measured by 1-year and multiple-year periods
12. r = .96 between multiple non-industrial accidents of Group B, 1930–1948 samples, as measured by 1-year and multiple-year periods
13. r = .95 between non-industrial accidents of Group A, 1930–1948 samples, and cases of illness from all causes, 1947–1948 samples
14. r = .93 between non-industrial accidents of Group B, 1930–1948 sample, and cases of illness from all causes, 1947–1948 sample

Table 11.4 shows a nearly perfect correlation (r) between the age distribution of the various samples studied. A notable exception is the age distribution of multiple accidents in Groups A and B, (No. 8) where a low, though positive, correlation was obtained.

* r = coefficient of correlation.

TABLE 11.5

DIFFERENCES BETWEEN AGE DISTRIBUTION OF VARIOUS ACCIDENT SAMPLES

No.	$X^2 =$	*Significant* / X^2 *At 1% Level*	= Significance of Differences in Age Distribution of Accidents in
1	75.490	23.209	1930 Industrial Sample and 1930 Cincinnati Employed Population
2	174.260	20.090	1940 Industrial Sample and 1940 Cincinnati Employed Population
3	69.330	15.086	1946 Industrial Sample and 1946 Cincinnati Employed Population
4	1708.350	30.578	1930–1948 Non-Industrial Sample and Cincinnati Population, 1940 Census
5	1028.270	30.578	Significance of Difference in Age Distribution of Illness from all Causes, 1947–1948 Sample and Cincinnati Population, 1940 Census
			Significance of Difference in Age Distribution of Multiple Accidents in
6	103.490	26.217	Non-Industrial Group A and Industrial Sample
7	131.510	23.209	Non-Industrial Group B and Industrial Sample
8	217.270	27.688	Non-Industrial Groups A and B, 1930–1948 Sample
9	141.400	29.141	Males of Group A and Males of Group B
10	146.340	30.578	Females of Group A and Females of Group B
11	55.440	30.578	Group A and Population of Cincinnati, 1940 Census
12	270.110	30.578	Group B and Population of Cincinnati, 1940 Census

TABLE 11.6

DIFFERENCES BETWEEN AGE DISTRIBUTION OF VARIOUS ACCIDENT SAMPLES

No.	$X^2 =$	$\dfrac{Significant}{X^2 \text{ At } 1\% \text{ Level}} =$	Significance of Excess of Multiple Accidents in Group B as Compared to Group A
13	96.960	6.635	Total Group B as compared to Total Group A
14	57.640	6.635	Males of Group B as compared to Males of Group A
15	43.280	6.635	Females of Group B as compared to Females of Group A
16	21.417	6.635	Males of 1948 Industrial Sample as compared to Females
17	12.346	6.635	Males of 1946 Industrial Sample as compared to Females
			Significance of Differences in Accident Rate at Various Ages Compared to the General or Working Population of Cincinnati
18	8.320	6.635	Decrease in Per cent of Accidents at age 10–14 in Group A
19	45.217	6.635	Increase in Per cent of Accidents at age 10–14 in Group B
20	8.777	6.635	Increase in Per cent of Accidents at age 20–24 in 1946 Industrial Sample
21	14.376	6.635	Increase in Per cent of Accidents at age 25–34 in 1946 Industrial Sample

TABLE 11.7

DIFFERENCES BETWEEN AGE DISTRIBUTION OF VARIOUS ACCIDENT SAMPLES

No.	Critical Ratio	Increase in Per cent of Accident Rate at Various Ages
22	4.77	Ages 5–9 in Males of Group B as compared to Group A
23	4.70	Ages 5–9 in Males and Females of Group B as compared to Group A
24	9.54	Ages 20–24 in Non-Industrial Samples, 1930–1948
25	2.09	Ages 35–39 in Males of Group A
26	1.67	Ages 45–49 in Males of Group A
		Excess in Per cent of Multiple Accidents in
27	13.11	1930–1948 Industrial Sample as Compared to Non-Industrial Sample
28	14.89	1930–1948 Industrial Sample as Compared to Group A
29	8.01	1930–1948 Industrial Sample as Compared to Group B
30	6.07	Group B as Compared to Group A

Tables 11.5, 11.6 and 11.7 show that the differences obtained in these studies are statistically significant and that they could not have occurred by chance more than once in one hundred times. The only exceptions are in Numbers 25 and 26, where the differences are not statistically significant.

TABLE 11.8

DIFFERENCE BETWEEN AGE DISTRIBUTIONS OF 1930, 1940 AND 1946 INDUSTRIAL ACCIDENTS AND THE EMPLOYED POPULATION OF CINCINNATI (U. S. CENSUS)

	1930 Industrial Accidents				1940 Industrial Accidents				1946 Industrial Accidents		
Age	Observed	Expected	Difference	Age	Observed	Expected	Difference	Age	Observed	Expected	Difference
15–19	42	29	+13	15–19	83	46	+37	15–25	349	283	+66
20–24	72	59	+13	20–24	192	139	+53	25–34	468	393	+75
25–29	82	54	+28	25–34	402	293	+109	35–44	338	341	–3
30–34	65	48	+17	35–44	235	256	–21	45–54	222	284	–62
35–39	59	50	+9	45–54	118	210	–92	55–64	119	168	–49
40–44	33	43	–10	55–59	40	70	–30	65+	32	58	–26
45–49	19	36	–17	60–64	24	51	–27				
50–54	13	31	–18	65–74	17	38	–21				
55–59	11	23	–12	75+	...	3	–3				
60–64	3	17	–14								
65–69	2	10	–8								
Total	401	400			1111	1109			1528	1527	

X² = 75.49

X² = 23.209 at the 1% level of significance

X² = 174.26

X² = 20.090 at the 1% level of significance

X² = 69.33

X² = 15.086 at the 1% level of significance

From this study the conclusion was reached that the age distribution in these industrial accidents differs significantly from the age distribution of the employed population of Cincinnati as measured.

TABLE 11.9

DIFFERENCE BETWEEN AGE DISTRIBUTIONS OF THE 1930–1948 NON-INDUSTRIAL
ACCIDENTS AND THE CINCINNATI POPULATION (1940 CENSUS)

Age	Observed	Expected	Difference
0–4	682	491	+191
5–9	679	491	+188
10–14	577	562	+ 15
15–19	754	610	+144
20–24	1175	657	+518
25–29	967	681	+286
30–34	716	673	+ 43
35–39	682	634	+ 48
40–44	472	602	−130
45–49	416	578	−162
50–54	283	507	−224
55–59	196	412	−216
60–64	145	349	−204
65–69	74	277	−203
70–74	58	198	−140
75+	45	198	−153
Total	7921	7920	

$X^2 = 1708.350$

$X^2 = 30.578$ at the 1% level of significance

From this the conclusion is reached that the age distribution in these non-industrial accidents differs significantly from the age distribution of the Cincinnati population as measured.

CHAPTER FIVE

THE ACCIDENT SYNDROME

THE term "syndrome" almost has been preempted by the medical profession in descriptions of clinical disease states. So employed, the term "syndrome" is applied to recurrence of signs and/or symptoms that appear with fair regularity, although it is not necessary that every constituent of a syndrome always exist. Were the need to arise, it is possible that no fewer than fifty named clinical syndromes might be assembled. As just one example, "Banti's Syndrome" or "Symptom Complex"—"enlarged spleen, hypochromic anemia and leukopenia, often with cirrhosis and ascites." This syndrome is characteristic of congestive splenomegaly.

Syndromes may be recognized wholly apart from medicine and are descriptive of any regular or nearly regular recurrences in a series.

In the instance of the accident syndrome, it becomes desirable to set forth that it represents no purely clinical recurrences. Within this syndrome the clinical features stand out in striking fashion and may constitute the essence of the syndrome, but otherwise there are features scarcely to be linked with medicine or only indirectly so. Thus the detonating situation or trigger episode in itself is apart from medicine but constitutes an essentiality in the syndrome.

A syndrome is not the equivalent of an equation. Never may it be urged that of the units that comprise the accident syndrome $A + B + C =$ accident with or without injury. Rather, acceptance should be extended to the factual that $A + B + C$, or some other combination such as $C + D$, creates a situation favorable to the occasion of an accident with or without injury. The units that comprise the accident syndrome reduced to the fewest possible descriptive terms are presented in graph form as the Frontispiece.

UNIVERSAL RISK

One constant in the accident syndrome is universal risk. One of the certainties of life is that at all times every person lives in continual peril. At any moment, any person may be struck by a stray bullet; his eyes might be hit by a flying particle on the street; he might be bitten by an angry or rabid dog. Even his bed might collapse with ensuing injury. This universal risk may not be the same for all ages. At the moment of birth there is the peril that normal breathing may not be achieved. In old age there is the prospect of cardiac accident from even reasonable exertion. The fractured hip from a minor fall is a threat to the aged—little known to youth. There are universal risks sometime imperiling all, but sometime identified only with special periods of life. More often than not, the universal risk is associated with that ten per cent or twenty per cent of accidents wholly deriving from fortuitous circumstances. Chiefly, the universal risk becomes a part of the accident syndrome because of fear of injury. Many an accident is brought about because of a state of mind induced by the knowledge that danger exists. The simplest exemplification may be associated with over-nailing in the building of some structure where two nails might serve safety, but in apprehension beyond worry, six nails are deemed better and thus the wood is destroyed. A nervous, jumpy, nagging passenger in an automobile may so upset the otherwise reliable driver to the point of accident when ordinarily no accident would have appeared. Dread of accident thus becomes a consideration in the causation of accidents.

IRREGULAR ADDITIONAL RISK INCIDENT TO PHYSICAL IMPAIRMENT

Not on the main line of this exposition of the accident syndrome is the side issue of the influence of physical defection. No carefully devised argument is necessary to the acceptance of the physical handicap as a contributory factor to accident causation, but this is not invariably so. With adequate motivation or special effort, the physically handicapped may compensate for his impairment and frequently has fewer accidents, on equal exposure, than those not so afflicted. The unwary might be tempted to include mental defection as being closely akin to the physical. By design, all functional mental deviation is reserved for another grouping. Without debate deafness, blindness, color blindness, amputation, crippling of any type serves accident occurrence, although this is not a necessity or a regularity.

Apart from these obvious handicaps, others that attract less attention and not to be regarded as true physical defections contribute to an increased prospect of injury. Thus, individuals whose stature reaches six feet and two inches and above are hampered beyond commonplace recognition in automobile driving. Because of their height, their line of vision precludes the ready observation of overhead traffic signals and a current practice of tinting windshields in a diminishing density downward is such as to place the line of vision of the tall driver well into the densely colored section, thereby introducing increased exposure to reduced visibility over the average driver. Likewise, the exceptionally short individual is differently handicapped in some instances through inability easily to manipulate pedals. At the extremes of stature, individuals are also frequently handicapped in the use of work benches, tools, machinery, household utensils, furniture, entrances, etc.

The best example of the influence of physical impairment may be found in connection with those persons who are diabetics who may pass into coma or near coma as a result of hyperinsulinism, or those other persons under the influence of such drugs as marijuana or benzedrine. It might be argued that the effects of alcoholism fall into this same category, justification for which is admitted, but by design all functional mental disturbances foremostly are allocated to a following sphere embracing mental maladjustment and irresponsibility.

Less obvious in this situation of physical handicap is the impact of such handicap upon the mental outlook and behavior of those so afflicted. Such persons may not have undergone mental rehabilitation to the point of full adjustment to the new life situation. However, all such must be transferred in this epitomized presentation from the physical into that oncoming section devoted to maladjustment to the personal environment. In brief, it is the immediate intent to accord to physical defection a place—albeit a side place—in this accident syndrome arrangement.

ABNORMAL PHYSICAL ENVIRONMENT

Not always is it possible to thrust into the province of the fully fortuitous those accidents brought about by abnormal environmental circumstances. By some it might be contended that in the presence of an accident, an abnormal environment without exception exists although possibly only a momentary affair. This does not follow since it may be believed that many individuals are poorly adjusted to normal environments.

When an automobile driver is near blinded by the bright headlights of an oncoming vehicle, that is not fortuity, although the affront arising is not something within the control of the driver in the first instance. A long listing of items of that character continually contribute to the occurrence of accidents. A number of obvious examples are now mentioned: Noise, startle—as from lightning—, extremes in weather, downpour, upsetting odors, poor ventilation, occupational or vocational hazards, etc. It has been demonstrated earlier in this text that with regularity increased numbers of accidents occur during hot months. It may be insisted that these are the months of increased outdoor activities, sports, increased travel with attending congestion, longer daylight hours and all such. This may be granted, but the rejoinder is that in industry under identical mechanical conditions attending employment, accident frequency also rises in hot months. Readily it may be shown that in the extremes of hot weather, death rates from diseases mount, chiefly involving the aged but not wholly limited to those decades. It may be inferred as is axiomatic, that extreme high temperatures exact a toll of all persons, but culminating in death only for the few. In the southwest on a recent occasion, a sudden blinding sandstorm appeared making safe driving impossible and the suddenness afforded no opportunity to appraise the state of the safety of the road shoulder. One driver in uncertainty merely stopped in dilemma, but before any conclusion as to action could be reached, the car was struck by a truck coming from behind damaging both and blocking the road. Within a matter of a few minutes, fourteen cars successively plowed into one another and six deaths occurred. Readily enough this happening may be labeled an "act of God" and perhaps fortuity alone is the domain into which the entire catastrophe is to be relegated.

It becomes difficult under some circumstances to demark between universal risk and abnormal environments. An example may be found in a grade railroad crossing. That spot constitutes a perilous environment, but the risks entailed, while common enough, are not universal. Many persons suffer no exposure to grade crossings and many such intersections have lost their danger through over and underpasses. A worker in a garage repeatedly may be exposed to carbon monoxide. That gas is almost universal in its existence but little exists in concentrations that threaten those exposed. The coming of an unpredictable hailstorm may provide immediate danger to those caught in the open and certainly represents an unfavorable environment but is of such a rarity as not to be labeled a universal risk.

Without debating such issues, it becomes possible to raise many questions as to the significance of unexpected alteration in the environment. It is not easy to relegate such events to any exact place in the diagrammatic presentation of the accident syndrome.

MALADJUSTMENT AND IRRESPONSIBILITY

Of the several components of the accident syndrome, mental maladjustment and irresponsibility are the core. It is such maladjustment that unfailingly thrusts a portion of accident causation into clinical medicine. It is this territory that holds the greatest promise in the further substantial reduction in accidents now that conventional mechanical and educational devices have reached a plateau or at best, a gentle slope. It is manifest that no person constantly and completely is adjusted to his environment or himself. Even the occasional and transient maladjustment in the most stable of persons is conducive to accident. In a high percentage of individuals, maladjustments are frequent, often severe, often prolonged and often a continuing part of life.

The genesis of an accident without injury, due to transient maladjustment in a "normal" individual, may be aptly illustrated with a recent occurrence involving M. S. Many are familiar with the difficulties encountered in driving one of the large automobiles through the narrow garage doors of the older houses. In the present instance, the maneuver called for a skillful sharp turn and for approaching the entrance in a straight line. The driver always handled the situation with the skill and dispatch that comes with frequent repetition and many years of experience. Power steering and a spacious yard-way made it an effortless task.

On a Saturday night, the driver returned home from the theater, mildly reflective and a bit unhappy and disturbed by the play he had seen. The night was dark and dreary and the driver's mood was now somewhat in tune with the elements, although shortly before he had been completely at peace with himself and the world. Almost mechanically he pressed a button on the instrument panel of his car which opened the automatic garage door. Only after he was half-way inside the garage did he suddenly realize that the car was diagonal to the entrance and that he would have to retrack and make a fresh start. Instead of simply backing out in the same manner as he came in, he made a clumsy turn of the wheel, so that the car was now firmly wedged against one side of the door-way. It became apparent that to prevent damage to the vehicle and the door frame, he would have to get out of the car and appraise the direction of the wheels, the exact distribution of available clearance, etc. This was not done because it would have required removing his overcoat for a tight squeeze out of a narrowed passage-way. Only after the car was substantially damaged with some additional maneuvering was the original impulse to get out and inspect carried out and extrication of the vehicle was achieved without further damage.

By retracing the discernible factors in the development of this accident, it can be readily seen that the mishap had its origin in a mild and transient emotional strain which temporarily induced preoccupation, impaired perception, blunted good judgment and hampered proper coordination of movements. Under slightly different circumstances, the driver might have failed to notice a traffic light or to negotiate a curve; again he might have struck a pedestrian, collided with an oncoming vehicle, etc. Under the latter conditions or with a more intense upsurge of feelings, the ensuing accident easily might have resulted in serious bodily injury, severe property damage or worse.

The variations in the manner of occurrence of accidents are legion, while the basic principles involved are relatively few. The above illustration represents a slow-motion version of the sequence of events in the genesis of one accident. Ordinarily, the factors involved are more complex and the sequences are greatly accelerated and overlapping.

The main psychological or physiological elements that increase the probability of accidents in maladjusted persons are anxiety, fear, worry, guilt, hostilities, emotional and psychosexual conflicts, early exposure to aggression, overauthoritative parents or parent figures, broken homes, frustration, inadequacies of youth, rejection and fatigue. Clearly these stresses may derive from home life, occupation and community impacts.

It has proved possible to assemble no fewer than two hundred and fifty different factors contributing to maladjustment and accidents. The majority of these are purely mental, but numerous ones relate to mental states imposed by physical, environmental circumstances. It is inexpedient here to introduce any such long listing as two hundred and fifty. From that listing a few are presented to indicate the trend of the compilation:

> Aggressiveness
> Anger
> Attention getting ("show-off") tendencies
> Being easily offended
> Bereavement
> Boredom
> Competitiveness with inability to bear being outdone
> Deterioration from alcohol
> Deterioration from drugs
> Discontent
> Distraction
> Domestic strife
> Domination by strong drives to overcome opposition
> Excitement
> Faulty judgment of speed and distance
> Feelings of inferiority
> Feelings of superiority
> Frequently in conflict with authority
> Frustration
> Guilt feelings
> Hostility
> Impaired neuromuscular coordination
> Impairment of sensation

Impulsiveness
Indecision
Inexperience
Insecurity
Lack of attention to job at hand
Lonesomeness
Loss of parents
Love of power
Low order of judgment
Neurotic tendencies: anxiety, fear, depression, obsessions and compulsions
Overactivity
Personal conflicts
Preoccupation
Rashness in action
Rebelliousness
Resentment
Restlessness
Sexual abnormalities
Tendency to take chances or risks
Unconscious need for punishment (self-injury)
Unwillingness to accept monotony or routine, etc.

It is impossible fully to disassociate these mental factors from the more physical items contributing to the total. While the desire is to segregate for immediate purposes the mental factors listed, it readily becomes apparent that their significance is modified by such physical states or circumstances as youth, the male sex, excessive heat or cold, certain hours of the day, speed, haste, inexperience, recent previous accidents, faulty lighting, noise and startle.

Taking as a single example, "noise," no extended argument is in order to impose the recognition that disturbing noise even for stable persons may become a tremendous agent provocative of mental responses conducive to injury.

The major portion of this book is directed to these maladjustments as leading to accidents with or without injury and further is directed to the assertion that all too little exploration has been accorded this area in efforts further to reduce the incidence of accidents.

THE TRIGGER EPISODE

The readily discernible portion of the accident syndrome is the "trigger" event—the fire that burns, the nail stepped upon, the cinder in the eye, the bullet penetrating the body. In the instance of some ten per cent or fifteen per cent of accidental injuries, the trigger event is in itself an entity. None of the other constituents of the accident syndrome, save that of universal risk, is demonstrable. Then in a measure the term "trigger episode" is unwarranted, since in no degree are there antecedent factors, although behavior in the midst of the immediate accident excitant frequently relates to the injury or further injury or the severity of the injury. In the contemplation of the remaining eighty-five per cent of accidents, the trigger episode is but the expected outcome of the operation of all the antecedent factors comprising the accident syndrome. To the psychiatrist or psychologist the trigger event may become relatively unimportant, since the prospective victim of accidental mishap somewhat invariably will reach some accident culminator. The maladjusted individual ready for an accident may find his trigger episode anywhere—either in the home, at work, on the street or otherwise. Thus, that which is of tremendous importance to the uninitiated appraiser, becomes relatively unimportant to the psychiatrist or the psychologist.

It now becomes evident that the trigger episode in the majority of accidents is but the detonator of a far more powerful surcharge of etiologies. Less informed appraisers may fail to detect maladjustment in the presence of an accident that to them appears to be wholly fortuitous. Faced with the eventuality of an accident in which the trigger mechanism was a blown out automobile tire, they are prone to rate the occurrence as entirely a completeness within itself and without the influences of contributory factors. Better delineated, it may prove possible to detect lack of proper judgment as to the jeopardy of worn tires, the willingness to take chances or risks, speed or faulty judgment of speed or distances, an unconscious need for punishment, unwillingness to accept responsibility for routine precaution, rashness and other such possible contributions. With occasional exception, it may be contended that a blowout in a long used tire always reflects maladjustment on the part of the driver to the requirements of good judgment in the operation of a dangerous vehicle. An example less exhibitive of the workings of the accident syndrome is the hunter shot by his companion in the quest for the quarry. Without regard for the companion who may have to face his own shortcomings, rarely is the victim fully attended by the fortuitous. While the coroner's inquest may lead to a verdict of "death by accidental gunfire," a precise appraisal may be expected to reveal all manner of acts related to improper adjustment to the environmental picture. If all were known, there might be recorded rashness, failure to observe elementary hunting precautions, over-competitiveness, "show-off" tendencies, an urge to take undue risks, excitement, alcoholism, hurry, superiority, non-conformity and all such. Carried to the ultimate, it could be asserted that poor judgment is indicated by every hunter who enters a hunting area in which jeopardy is the rule and escape unharmed, the fortuity.

Similarly approached a legion of accidents varying in characteristics from A to Z may be shown to result more from the background than from the trigger episode. Notwithstanding all this, the detonation is to be accepted as a necessary evil element in the constellation of affairs that explode into the accident with or without injury.

BEHAVIOR IN THE PRESENCE OF THE TRIGGER MECHANISM

The pattern of behavior of the individual when confronted with a sudden decision or danger will frequently determine whether the forces set in motion will eventuate in a near miss or in an accident. Occasionally behavior in the presence of the trigger may also determine the occurrence of injury as well as its severity. In a schematic presentation of the accident syndrome, the behavior in the presence of the trigger mechanism should be related chiefly to the antecedent maladjustment of the individual rather than precisely linked to the trigger itself.

In event of an accident the severity of an injury is not always determined by the trigger episode, although often it is. For example, in the instance of a person's clothing being ignited, one person prudently will seek to smother the flame by wrapping himself or causing himself quickly to be wrapped in an overcoat or nearby blanket. Another person in stark panic aimlessly may run and thus pave the way for death or severe damage. In another instance in the presence of a small laceration, the victim may elect to ignore the injury, but the wary and knowing individual intelligently will seek medical care, thereby avoiding further injury through infection. In a third instance in the case of a plane crash in the arctic region, one pilot cautiously and promptly will dig himself into a nearby snowbank and will protect himself against the prospect of freezing. The scatterbrained pilot, with or without injury, may wander aimlessly until exhausted and freeze to death. Through these three responses is indicated what is meant by behavior after the trigger circumstance. Clearly such behavior, at least in part, is determined not by the immediate exigencies, but by long antecedent adjustment, training or experience here categorized in the vernacular as adjustment to one's life situation. Manifestly, proper behavior grows out of a background of intelligent grasp of potentialities. Conversely, faulty behavior, in a measure, stems from just the opposite—maladaptations that precisely pave the way for disastrous mishaps.

THE PROSPECTIVE ACCIDENT WITH OR WITHOUT INJURY

Confronted with some or all of the circumstances conducive to accident causation, it does not follow that an accident with or without injury is inevitable. Under observable conditions, oftentimes it appears near to the miraculous that an accident does not occur. When personal injury comes about and particularly promptly after that injury, the victim, in a high percentage of the total, is in a state favorable to the detection of the background of events or circumstances that paved the way for the accident. Nothing that the physician may do at that time has any bearing upon the accident at hand, but an outstanding opportunity exists for the detection of maladjustment and thus some measure of prophylaxis against future mishaps may exist. It is at this period that the provocations of maladjustment become surface phenomena, although that statement not always is valid. At once a dilemma arises. While the average physician may take advantage of the many disclosures that may appear, rarely is he equipped with such psychiatric training as to warrant any deep probing into the patient's background. In truth, witless probings may pave the way for added resentments and hostilities directed to the physician and traumatic neuroses may have their initiation. On the other hand, in the presence of trivial or minor injuries, there exists no obvious reason why the psychiatrist or psychologist should be injected into the situation. In this dilemma the most practical procedure may reside in the physician's mere recording the spontaneous declarations indicative of previous disturbing maladjustments. What may take place during this period and in particular if the patient be hospitalized, is now reviewed with an eye to the components of the accident syndrome in the contribution to the mishap.

As a frequency it comes about that the accident victim as a patient is accorded less humane consideration than some other classes of patients. Too often the attitude on the part of physicians and nurses is one of relative aloofness and the willingness to stigmatize, predicated upon the assumption that this class of patients is less deserving of sympathy in that their troubles in some measure were brought upon themselves. The degree of this aloofness certainly will not reach the point of neglect and chiefly is expressed in lack of sympathy. Inevitably this serves to wall off the patient and thus deprives the physician of information that well might contribute to the prevention of future accidents.

The patient may reveal to the physician his previous aggressive tendencies that might have been a factor in the accident causation through continued aggression directed toward the physician, the nurses and all about him. If this projection of feelings of hostility and guilt onto the physician may be avoided and a position of confidence arises, the physician without probing may become the ready outlet for the victim's draining of feelings of resentment, fear, hatred, through endless variation to the end result of full delineation of the unfavorable contributory factors in the accident's causation. Not only recent malhappenings become items voiced in sympathetic conversations, but long-forgotten, painful experiences may float to the foreground of consciousness during the period of necessary treatment. It is during this time that spontaneously the patient may make clear unfavorable relations within his environment, the source of his guilt, the causes of hostility toward employer, foreman, fellow worker, wife, children, parents, in-laws and on and on within the totality of some two hundred and fifty factors earlier mentioned, some ones of which play a role in eighty-five per cent of all accidents.

More often than not, the willingness to pour out the background of difficulties may be extended to the nurse to a degree greater than for the physician. The all-wise and sympathetic nurse may play a tremendous role in the determination of the factors of disturbance that brought about the injury and thus becomes the natural ally of the physician in these activities, hopefully directed to the avoidance of future accidents.

Since the immediate and past emotional states of a person frequently play a determining part in the causation of the accident, these should be given due consideration by the treating physician. In fact, to a judicious degree they become one of the objectives of treatment. In nearly all accidents which are related to personality factors, there is a fleeting breakdown in the adequate control of coordinated or integrated voluntary behavior. This breakdown may take place in one of three areas. It may be due to faulty perception, faulty reasoning and interpretation or faulty mechanisms for discharging excess emotional tensions—chronic or acute instinctual as well as subconscious ideational tensions.

Some accidents are motivated by unconscious thought processes that cannot find an outlet in some motor behavior because of repression. This type of accident has a specific "meaning" and can be interpreted by appropriate analytical methods in the same manner as other psychoneurotic symptoms. From this point of view the accident is a neurotic symptom and represents an abnormal mechanism for relieving excess psychic tension. Whether the accident is due to specific psychopathology or merely to a momentary breakdown of normal adaptive defense mechanisms for dealing with stressful life situations, the accident should be considered as a sign that the patient was either under temporary or chronic emotional strain prior to the accident and should be treated accordingly.

Whatever the state of the patient prior to the accident, there is a period of anxiety or fear following the accident which in turn stimulates a new set of defenses. The usual defenses against anxiety, in accidents as in general illness, are:

> A denial reaction—the patient minimizes, reduces or denies the importance of the injury, refuses medical attention, denies the existence of pain, etc.

Aggressive behavior—the patient may put on a front, exaggerate his symptoms, put the blame for the injury on someone else, accuse the physician or others in attendance of neglect or mistreatment, etc.

After the initial phase of post-injury anxiety and the immediate defense reaction which follows, most patients soon accept the injury as a fact and enter what may be called in injury as in illness, the phase of being ill. The patient regresses to more primitive patterns of behavior and a number of benefits or "secondary gains" accrue. He becomes self-centered and body conscious (narcissistic regression) his needs become simpler, he becomes more dependent and there is a reduced sense of responsibility. The patient may become demanding, selfish and intolerant and there may be outbursts of temper, jealousy, obstinancy, apathy, disinterest and hypochondriasis.

Since accident patients are frequently under apparent concealed or subconscious emotional strain, it follows that the physician should provide the patient with adequate relationship therapy, with an opportunity for verbal ventilation, with insight therapy or psychiatric consultation, as the particular case might require. The occasions of the critical care of the injury and subsequent dressings or treatments should be recognized as the golden opportunity for helping the patient rid himself of the excess accumulation of psychological or emotional stresses in the manner most suitable to his needs and personality. The interest in the patient should be continued beyond the surgical emergency and even beyond the complete healing of the wound and he should be considered completely cured only when the physician is satisfied that the patient is no longer under pressure of emotional strain.

By no means does it follow from this discussion that only after one accidental injury and during the period of treatment therefor, resides the occasion for the detection of maladjustment and thus paving the way for effort in the prevention of future unwanted events. Still, it may be emphasized that during that time much may be assembled that provides support to the thesis of this book. Mental maladjustment is at the present time the major domain in the ultimate etiology of accidents. If additional major reductions in the frequency of accidents are to be achieved, the elimination of mental maladjustment becomes the heart of newness in safety programs. It is at this point that the physician rather than the engineer enters and thus accident prevention more than ever before is thrust, however much unwanted, into clinical medicine. The demand is for a wider and more enlightened participation on the part of all those who treat the injured, especially general physicians, industrial physicians, pediatricians, orthopedists and surgeons who will in turn avail themselves of the special skills of psychiatrists and psychologists whenever the occasion demands.

It is the earnest intent of this chapter, indeed the entire book, to provide conviction that the usual accident derives from mental maladjustment, that this maladjustment is the product of many scores of causative factors and that regardless of teeming variations, there arises a constellation of events or circumstances that comprise a syndrome—the accident syndrome.

CHAPTER SIX

ACCIDENT PRONENESS (55)

The finding that a small percentage of the population is involved in most of the accidents variously has been interpreted and has led to a considerable amount of misdirected effort. It is being taught in the schools and preached over the air and in the press that fifteen per cent of the population is responsible for eighty-five per cent of all accidents, and that all we need to do to solve the accident problem is to detect and cure this small group of people. The question arises whether this "fifteen per cent of the population that suffers eighty-five per cent of all the accidents" is a fixed group of accident-prone individuals or whether it is merely a statistical concept of an ever-changing population.

The British Medical Research Council writes that there is a tendency for those who have an undue number of accidents in one period to have an undue number of accidents in all subsequent periods "each hour of the day, each day of the week, each month of the year, and each subsequent year." Again, from the Transactions of the 35th National Safety Congress: "A relatively small number of employees account for the great majority of industrial injuries. These employees are so highly susceptible to accidents that they cannot avoid having them regardless of how anxious they may be to do so. . . . They are the persons who are affecting the accident rate to the greatest degree. In fact, the elimination of the accident-proneness of these . . . . employees (eight per cent) would result in a forty-five per cent decrease in total minor injuries."

Such is the prevailing view in the literature and the generally accepted working basis in the field of safety and accident prevention.

The writer's clinical experience and studies do not support this view. Analysis of twenty-seven thousand consecutive industrial accidents, coming from a great variety and number of industrial plants, and of eight thousand consecutive non-industrial accidents, indicates that:

1. The tendency to have accidents is, in the main, a phenomenon that passes with age, decreasing steadily after reaching a peak at the age of twenty-one. The accident rate at the age of twenty to twenty-four, in both our industrial and non-industrial series, is two and a half times higher than at the age of forty to forty-four, four times higher than at the age of fifty to fifty-four, and nine times higher than at the age of sixty to sixty-five.
2. Most accidents are due to the increased liability to accidents of youth. Seventy percent of the non-industrial accidents occurred before the age of thirty-five and nearly fifty per cent before the age of twenty-four.
3. Men are significantly more liable to accidents than women, the ratio of male to female accidents being two to one in the non-industrial series and apparently even higher in the industrial series.
4. Most accidents (seventy-four per cent) are due to relatively infrequent solitary experiences of large numbers of individuals (eighty-six per cent). These figures were identical for the industrial as well as for the non-industrial series, and remained constant for nearly every year of a twenty-year period.
5. Those who suffer injuries year after year, over a period of three years (three to five per cent), account for a relatively small percentage of all the accidents (one-half of one per cent).
6. Irresponsible and maladjusted individuals are significantly more liable to have accidents than responsible and normally adjusted individuals.

From the foregoing it can be computed that, on the basis of age and sex distribution alone, a small percentage of a given population could account for most of the accidents. Simple chance is, of course, also a factor in the unequal distribution of accidents. The presence in any population of an undue number of highly "accident-prone" individuals would naturally accentuate the unequal distribution due to the factors of age, sex and chance. Our studies indicate that, when the period of observation is sufficiently long, most accidents occur in individuals with a low degree of proneness, and that the relatively small percentage of the population that contributes a disproportionate number of accidents is essentially a shifting group, with new persons constantly falling in and out of the group. The excessive liability to accidents in youth seems to disappear with age and, in most of the highly "accident-prone" individuals, with learning, with physiological and psychological adaptation, or with the development of more adequate psychological defenses.

Clinical experience suggests that in the course of a life span almost any normal individual under emotional strain or conflict may become temporarily "accident-prone" and suffer a series of accidents in fairly rapid succession. Most persons, however, find solutions to their problems, develop defenses against their emotional conflicts, and drop out of the highly accident-prone group after a few hours, days, weeks or months. Some persons remain highly "accident-prone" throughout life, with or without lapses of years of freedom from the accident habit. The latter are the truly "accident-prone" individuals. They contribute, however, only a relatively small percentage of all the accidents.

This point of view is not without support in the literature. Vernon states that accident frequency usually decreases with age; also, ". . . the accident-proneness of various individuals is not a fixed quality, but is liable to be affected by any and every change in their bodily condition. This condition is influenced by external changes of environment as well as by internal changes of physical and mental health." Johnson in an intensive study conducted for the U. S. Government, concluded that there exist two groups of accident-prone individuals; those who are now young and those who have had an unusually high rate of accidents in the past. Horn, in a study of ten thousand aircraft pilots who have had two or more accidents in the air, shows that a pilot is much more likely to have another accident within thirty days of his first one—but the probability that he will have another accident decreases markedly as time passes. Dunbar concluded that the accident habit is not necessarily a fixed quality. Cobb found that vehicle operators .... "who are accident-repeaters in one period tend to regress toward the average of the group in another period."

Brown and Ghiselli, in a study of the accident experience of ninety-three trolley car and motor coach operators, found that the coefficient of correlation of the number of accidents sustained in odd and even months over an eighteen-month period, showed a wide range of variation, from 1.9 to 0.80 with an average of 0.40. From this, the authors conclude that "accident proneness as a general trait of the individual has not been substantiated."

In 1929, in an analysis of half a million accidents, Heinrich demonstrated a fixed relationship between accidents with injury and accidents without injury, as well as between major (lost-time) and minor injuries. Similar accidents, Heinrich states, may produce minor or major injuries or no injury at all. In a unit group of three hundred and thirty similar accidents, three hundred result in no injury, twenty-nine in minor injuries and one in a major injury. On the basis of these studies and an estimated annual toll of ten million lost-time injuries, there are, roughly, three billion accidents and three hundred million minor injuries annually in the U.S.A.

Such an over-abundance of mishaps suggests that accidents are a common human characteristic. In our own experience there have been few individuals past the age of early childhood who have not had at least several minor injuries. Memory alone is a poor guide to the incidence of injury; patients will often deny previous injury when numerous scars on exposed areas obviously tell a different story. We therefore agree with Vernon that it is more nearly correct to speak of relative degrees of "accident-proneness," rather than of the presence or absence of proneness. The evidence presented is in sharp conflict with the prevailing theory that most accidents are sustained by a relatively small and fixed group of individuals.

SUMMARY

The currently accepted theory that most accidents are sustained by a small fixed group of "accident-prone" individuals is open to question. On the basis of clinical experience and studies, the author suggests that most accidents are due to relatively infrequent solitary experiences of large numbers of individuals. The total number of accidents suffered by those who injure themselves year after year, over a period of three or more years, is relatively small. The frequently observed unequal distribution of accidents appears, among other things, to be due to unequal liability to accidents on the basis of age and sex, to transient or prolonged states of physical, physiological or psychological stress, to chronic "accident-proneness" and to chance. The evidence indicates that if the period of observation is sufficiently long, the "small group of persons who are responsible for most of the accidents" is essentially a shifting group of individuals with new persons constantly falling in and out of the group. It seems to be more nearly correct to speak of varying degrees of "accident-proneness" rather than of the presence or absence of proneness.

CHAPTER SEVEN

PSYCHOLOGICAL FACTORS IN ACCIDENT CAUSATION AND PREVENTION

For the past two decades, accidents have ranked first among the causes of death in young men under the age of thirty-five. For the population as a whole, they now rank fourth among all causes of death (third for males) and third in the tables of incidence of illness. One hundred thousand persons meet violent death annually as a result of accidents; four hundred thousand sustain permanent impairment of body or limb; ten million suffer injuries resulting in one or more days of disability. The equivalent of a year's labor by a million men is lost annually to the nation as a result of injuries and the total annual cost of accidents now reaches the staggering sum of ten billion dollars.

The anxiety, the pain, and the mental anguish stirred up by accidents, the emotional disequilibrium into which many family groups are thrown as a result of accidents and their social and economic concomitants are also of extreme importance in this problem. Accidents often occur in a chain fashion, as if one accident carried with it the seed of, or acted as a trigger mechanism or as a sensitizing agent, for another accident in patient, family, friend or bystander. Proneness to multiple accidents tends to develop more frequently in patients with an early history of exposure to violence or tragedy; especially where there have been broken homes, family strife and accidental death or injury of parent or sibling.

The past four decades have been marked by an intensive investigation of the accident problem. Private industry, labor organizations and the states have spent millions and have mobilized the arts as well as the sciences in the cause of accident prevention. Safety has been stressed by press, pulpit and cinema and its precepts have been taught in the classroom. Courts of law have imposed heavy penalties for violation of rules of safety on the roads and in factories. The machinery and methods of industrial and agricultural production have been constantly improved so as to make it increasingly difficult to injure oneself. A sizable army of safety engineers has been devoting itself full time to the task of perfecting preventive measures. Recent advances in medical and surgical therapeutics have greatly reduced the morbidity and mortality rates of the injured. Definite progress has also been made in reducing the frequency and severity rates of accidents in industry. Yet viewing the accident problem as a whole, the practical achievements in the saving of life and limb have lagged behind the amount of effort expended. Obviously there must be some factor or factors which have slowed progress toward a substantial reduction in death and injury caused by accidents.

The exigencies of World War I provided the first serious incentive for the study of accidents, particularly for the study of environmental hazards in industry and their relation to the frequency and severity of injuries. The advent of the automobile, with the steady rise of sudden and violent death on the road, gave further impetus to the study of accidents.

The importance of environmental hazards in the etiology of accidents can be gauged from published statistics on the incidence of injury in the various industries. In 1949, the frequency rate of injury ranged from 2.14 injuries per 1,000,000 man-hours of work in the communications industry, to 47.72 in the lumber industry, with a frequency rate of 10.14 for all industries combined.

A great deal of useful information has become available as a result of continuing efforts to effect accident reduction through the elimination of environmental hazards. Gradually, it was learned that although the removal of hazards was a constant necessity, accidents frequently occur where environmental hazards are minimal or where they are difficult to control. It was furthermore discovered that the hazard as well as the accident is often a product of human failings, such as haste, speed, preoccupation or faulty judgment, and that these, in turn, are frequently related to states of emotional strain or conflict. As a result of these findings, increasing emphasis began to be placed on the relation of accidents to human behavior. With this change of emphasis, accident prevention took an abrupt turn in the direction of psychological and psycho-analytical explorations of the mind and personality of the accident patient.

A number of other important observations contributed to this change of emphasis:
1. Eighty to ninety per cent of all accidents, it was found, are traceable to something in the personality of the individual and only ten to fifteen per cent are truly fortuitous.
2. Under identical conditions of exposure and environment, some people have significantly more accidents than others.
3. Most accidents (fifty-five to one hundred per cent) are sustained by a relatively small per cent (fifteen to twenty-five per cent) of the population, the accident-prone.

ACCIDENT CAUSATION — IN REVIEW

Greenwood and Woods were the first to call attention to multiple accidents as an important factor in the incidence of injury in industry. Marbe called it the "accident habit" and provided statistical evidence that the probability of having accidents is greater in the person who has had previous accidents. Marbe also suggested that the personality factor has more significance than the type of occupation. Hildebrandt disclosed that personal conditions play a more important part in causing accidents than slow reactivity. The National Research Council, Rawson and others found that accident-prone individuals are accident-prone in any occupation. Heyman asserts that accident proneness, or predisposition, is the determining factor in human accidents. The past decade has witnessed a loud chorus of approval and general acceptance of the above views.

Greenwood and Woods concluded that "accident-proneness" is a measurable quality. This optimistic view of the measurability of "accident-proneness" has fallen short of realization; few of the multitude of tests which have been tried to date have proved to be more than of limited usefulness. Cobb, Johnson and others have shown that facts drawn from the best of all possible tests do not validate prediction concerning the performance of any individual. Clinical experience has shown that even a past history of repeated accidents is not an accurate indication of "accident-proneness." It was learned that the future accident experience of any individual cannot be foretold or predicted on the basis of a past history of repeated accidents unless adequate allowance is made for unusual exposure to hazards and a host of other factors.

Karl Menninger advanced the theory that certain accidents are unconsciously purposive. The body suffers damage as a result of circumstances which appear to be fortuitous but which, upon analysis, are found to fulfill specific unconscious tendencies of the victim. These accidents, according to Menninger, represent the capitalization of an opportunity for focal or total self-destruction by the death instinct. A sacrificial principle appears to be in operation and the motives in the accidents include the elements of aggression, punition and propitiation.

Flanders Dunbar and her group attempted to delineate the personality profile of the "accident-prone" individual, which would serve both accident prediction and accident prevention. Although they failed in both of these objectives, their work has had a great impact on the study of accidents and has led to a better understanding of the psychodynamics of certain types of accidents and of "accident proneness."

According to Dunbar, the behavior pattern of fracture patients is characterized by a striving for independence or autonomy in their relationship with authoritarian figures, an outward casualness about feelings and personal problems and a tendency toward impulsive action. At least one factor which predisposes to accidents, Dunbar contends, is this conflict between repressive authoritarian pressures and the striving toward independent behavior. By focusing their values on short term concrete experiences and by avoiding marked submission or domination in vocational and social roles, the fracture patients usually manage to minimize or avoid serious conflicts with authority. When these usual defenses of the fracture patient fail and he can find no satisfactory escape from his hostility and guilt, his aggressiveness breaks out in an impulse to punish both himself and those responsible for his frustration.

In the numerous studies that have followed those of Dunbar and Menninger, nearly every type of specific emotional conflict and nearly every shade of non-specific mental aberration has been implicated in the causation of accidents. The writer's own observations and studies tend to suport the findings of others that both primary and secondary psychological gain play a role in some accidents and that some accidents and injuries have symbolic significance to the individual.

It is quite evident that we have come a long way from the erstwhile prevailing concepts that all accidents are due to carelessness or that they are chance occurrences. The theory that most accidents are related to personality problems is a decided step forward and heralds the possibility of at least a partial solution of the accident problem. Personality deviations, however, are so universal, "accident-proneness" is so ill-defined, and the "accident-prone" group as a whole is so evanescent and elusive, that for practical purposes this newest hypothesis carries almost the same connotation of futility as the earlier concepts.

ACCIDENT PREVENTION

Among the major difficulties which prevent the translation of the newer psychological concepts of accident causation into practical preventive measures are: (1) A seemingly deep seated resistance to the relinquishment of the comfortable notion that accidents are fortuitous events. (2) Reluctance on the part of the accident patient to accept possible stigmatization as a mental or emotional deviant. (3) Inability or unwillingness of many psychiatrically unsophisticated minds, lay and professional alike, to accept some of the psychiatric principles involved. It is difficult for some individuals to comprehend such concepts as unconsciously purposive accidents, focal suicide, death instinct, repressive authoritarian pressure, castration anxiety etc. Many find such terms confusing, equivocal and even revolting. Despite the phenomenal progress in recent years, toward psychiatric sophistication, one is impressed by the magnitude of the residual undercover resistance towards modern psychiatric concepts.

It seems that if we are to deal more effectively with the accident problem, a new and more intensive educational effort will have to be devised, aimed primarily at the individual and reaching into all elements of the population. Since nearly all of the causative factors of accidents ultimately relate to the human factor, there is a need for more intensive research and more precise information about the mechanisms involved and about the interrelationships of the various accident factors. Of special interest are such matters as motivation, emotional stress, maladjustment to stressful life situations, certain physiological and metabolic factors, etc. For the purposes of study as well as prevention, it might be well to single out for special attention the young, the male, the maladjusted, the irresponsible, the chronically accident-prone of all ages and all other peak areas of accident causation by age, sex, season, hour of day, special hazard etc.

In educational and safety efforts, it might be well to emphasize that anyone under emotional strain may be as much of a menace to himself and to others while driving a car, at work, at play or in his home, as a person under the influence of alcohol. The relationship of accidents to such factors as insecurity, domestic strife, loss of parent and exposure to injury in parent or sibling also needs to be stressed.

There is also need for a wider awareness that even trivial injury may be an outward manifestation of an underlying emotional strain or conflict. Too often, in the case of minor injuries, the physician-patient relationship is that of an annoyed physician and an apologetic patient. A golden opportunity for psychological diagnosis and the application of preventive medical principles is thus passed up, unrecognized and unutilized, while the patient is cheerfully unloaded to the nurse or attendant for the application of a dressing.

While treating the injured, it might be well to remember that the accident patient is often a troubled individual who may be in need of sympathetic understanding and a bit of kindness. It cannot be overemphasized that the patient who merely gets his wounds dressed and is otherwise ignored or neglected, is more likely to develop traumatic or compensation neurosis and is also more likely to have another and perhaps more serious injury. The accident patient may, in reality, be seeking a supporting relationship which will relieve him of a stressful life situation which has become intolerable. Failure to relieve the emotional strain of the patient and to recognize the possible true significance, even of the most trivial of injuries, may eventuate in a series of accidents, one of which may well be serious or fatal.

When trying to uncover the possible psychogenic factors underlying an accident, a few principles may be of help. Probing and meaningful psychological interpretation are potentially dangerous tools and are best left to the psychiatrist. A great deal of useful diagnostic and therapeutic material will often come forth from the patient spontaneously, if given half a chance to unburden himself. A friendly, cheerful and sympathetic attitude, together with a genuine interest in the welfare of the patient as a worthwhile fellow human being, will usually break the ice and bring forth sufficient material for a working diagnosis.

To prevent the onset and to facilitate the treatment of traumatic and compensation neurosis, kindness must be tempered with firmness and thoroughness. The first contact with the patient is of utmost importance. A friendly sympathetic attitude on the part of the physician will usually dispel a patient's suspicion that the doctor may be part of the hostile environment. It may also serve to provide the patient with immediate psychological gains which can be of decisive prophylactic and therapeutic importance. There is the occasional patient whose feelings of guilt and need for punishment are so great that he will react adversely to a friendly, giving attitude on the part of the physician. This type of patient is strictly a psychiatric problem and should be treated as such.

A thorough physical examination, in addition to establishing the exact nature, extent and severity of the injury, will provide some additional beneficial psychological gains for the patient and will often help to set his potential claims within reasonable and realistic limits. The x-ray, being endowed with magic attributes in many lay minds, can serve as an effective tool to discourage the precipitation of a neurosis, especially if the x-ray examination is negative and is made soon after the injury. In the presence of a physician-patient relationship based on mutual repsect, firmness can be an effective adjunct to kindness and thoroughness in the prevention and treatment of traumatic and compensation neurosis.

While the frequency and severity rates of accidents in industry have declined during the past two decades, virtually no progress has been made in reducing the seventy to eighty per cent of the accidents which occur outside of industry. Progress in the reduction of accidents in small industry, which employs about sixty per cent of the working population, leaves much to be desired; while progress at reducing home accidents, which account for about fifty per cent of all the mishaps, is at a virtual standstill. In the meanwhile the spotlight has turned on the automobile accident. It may be of interest to note that automobile accidents have risen to the forefront among the various types of accidents without materially affecting the total number of accident injury, disability or fatality cases from all causes.

The mounting interest in automobile accidents stems from their alarming frequency in recent years. Rising public apprehension is especially justified in view of the annual toll of thirty-six thousand lives and the high rates of morbidity and permanent disability which result from these accidents. The increase in the frequency of automobile accidents is generally attributed to congestion on the roads, due to more numerous vehicles on inadequate highways. Of much greater importance, perhaps, is the poor quality of many of the new drivers. An unprecedented wave of prosperity and easy credit terms have combined to place motor cars in the hands of the worst "accident-makers"—the young, the maladjusted and the irresponsible. Thus the automobile—one of the great blessings and proud symbols of twentieth century civilization—is rapidly becoming a dreaded instrument of destruction.

This is the challenge which faces the student of the accident problem today. It should be met by more intensive research, by teams of safety engineers, psychologists, psychiatrists, physiologists and clinicians. Promising results may be obtained by: (1) Taking advantage of some of the knowledge gained in dealing with the accident problem in industry. (2) Utilizing the more recent advances in the study of accidents. (3) Submitting earlier studies to review in the light of present day experience and thinking. (4) Placing greater reliance on the clinical approach. (5) Conducting long-range integrated studies on large groups of hard-core accident repeaters. (6) Controlled epidemiological studies of accidents in various parts of the world. Such studies, as above outlined, should eventually lead to a more complete understanding of accident causation and to substantial accident reduction. To serve more immediate needs, various improvisations and adaptations to newly gained knowledge will have to suffice.

It should not be necessary nor would it be desirable at this juncture to spell out in any great detail a definitive program of accident prevention. When the true nature of the problem is properly understood, when the importance of accident reduction to the well-being of the nation and the individual is fully appreciated and public opinion is sufficiently aroused, there will undoubtedly emerge an accident prevention program capable of meeting the challenge. The search for a solution may follow traditional epidemiological lines and may concern itself with the well known triad of host, agent and environment. Following the generally successful examples of the popular movements for combatting tuberculosis, cancer, heart disease, poliomyelitis, diabetes—and recently alcoholism—the new approach to accident prevention should develop on a broad popular base, with the active cooperation and leadership of organized medicine.

It seems significant that although some ten million accident patients reach physicians' offices annually and thus constitute a sizeable portion of medical practice, it is about the only medical condition in which physicians rarely concern themselves with cause or prevention. It may also be worth noting that as of this late date, the subject of accidents cannot claim a scientific forum it may call its own. Accidents (not the surgical treatment of injuries) are seldom considered an appropriate topic for discussion at scientific medical meetings, are seldom included in the curriculum of medical schools and are rarely dignified by full fledged scientific investigations or sizeable grants.

As a long-range problem in public education and health, accidents in some respects share common ground with such other problems as juvenile delinquency, major crime, high divorce rate, alcoholism, drug addiction and social and economic maladjustment. In common with the others, many accidents represent a problem in poor mental hygiene, in defective moral and religious values, in faulty cultural standards or in the lack of ability readily to adjust to adverse life situations.

As a problem in safe practices, accident prevention faces a dilemma. Basically the concept of "safety" implies that accidents are preventable and that they are not fortuitous events. Yet repeatedly this implication is negated throughout life when we console our children, relatives and friends with such expressions as: "It was only an accident," "You really could not help it," or "Accidents will happen." To what extent is accident prevention hampered by such continued indoctrination that the individual bears no responsibility for his accidents? These and similar phrases no doubt are intended as expressions of sympathy, in conformity with our cultural mores. Nonetheless, their usage, especially during the early impressionable years of childhood, cannot but hinder the cause of accident prevention and should be abandoned. Similar consideration needs to be given the very term "accident," for in its most intended usage it no longer relates either to fortuity or triviality. Since its abandonment may not be considered practical, new meaning should be put into the term through intensive use of the educational process.

At the present juncture accident prevention could perhaps be served best if medical examinations were given to all persons with frequent accidents, to those who are under severe emotional strain, and to those who are engaged in hazardous pursuits. Medical examinations are especially indicated in the three main accident-producing groups—the young, the male, and the maladjusted, and where personal and family histories contain important accident-predisposing factors. The vast majority of those examined should benefit from the mere evaluation of their accident potential and the insight gained therefrom. Some may require a brief course of superficial therapy. Only a relatively few would require psychiatric help.

It need not be inferred from any of the aforesaid that accident prevention depends on reforming the human race. The objectives are quite modest: a more realistic approach, improved mental hygiene and additional aids for self-preservation.

CHAPTER EIGHT

THE INCIDENCE OF ACCIDENTS IN IRRESPONSIBLE AND MALADJUSTED INDIVIDUALS

ALL major investigations of the background from which the majority of accidents spring emphasize the peculiar significance of abnormal personality traits. Irresponsible, unreliable and maladjusted individuals constitute an outstanding reservoir of accident causation. In a just sense these individuals may be labeled "accident-prone," but throughout this text resistance has been introduced to the widely accepted concept that a small fixed proportion of the total population provide the victims of the majority of accidental events.

It was fully expected that among the individuals giving rise to this present series of thirty-five thousand consecutive accident records, a large number would warrant the label of "irresponsibility." Already in that chapter concerned with work materials has been mentioned a certain "Group B," the medical records pertaining thereto having been critically examined in regard to irresponsibility and maladjustment. By no means does it follow that this highly selected group contains all of the irresponsible characters, but this group does provide opportunity for comparison with other groups accepted as more stable. In iteration, it is observed that this group in the first instance was selected on the basis of the criterion of the non-payment of just medical charges in the absence of any apparent reason for such evasion. Ultimately, only the records which were certified as "uncollectible" were included in Group B. If there be any unfavorable criticism that this basis of selection is highly artificial, let it be recorded that the physician in ministering to members of this group and preparing records pertaining thereto, came to possess many other indications of unreliability, irresponsibility and maladjustment. However, segregation on their basis of financial negligence appeared to be fully justified from analysis of accidental experiences on comparison with Group A.

The records from Group B afforded abundant evidence of high frequency of family strife, broken homes, maltreatment of children, delinquency, alcoholism and legal entanglement. Twenty-five per cent of all the accidents in Group B were due to fights and other forms of aggressive behavior compared with only 15.5% of this type of accident in Group A. The patients of Group B also were notable for their frequent shifts in employment and residence. The bulk of the other non-industrial patients (Group A) were, by these same standards, more nearly normally adjusted and responsible. However, the members of this Group A were not as homogeneous as Group B, since many members were indigent and many known to be maladjusted who, no less, paid their medical bills. There was no appreciable difference in the size of the families of these groups.

A comparative study of the frequency of repeated or multiple accidents in Groups A and B showed that of all the accidents in Group B, 21.5% were multiple ones, as against 13.9% in Group A—an increase of fifty-four per cent in the frequency of multiple accidents in Group B over A. Nearly identical results were obtained when the numbers of patients with multiple accidents were compared instead of their accidents. The difference in the accident frequency of the two groups of patients was found to grow in almost geometric proportion, when the number of accidents per person increased from two, to three, or four and more; thus:

> In patients with two accidents each the excess accident frequency in Group B over A was only 1.18% to 1%.
> In patients with three accidents each the ratio became 2.29% to 1%.
> In patients with four or more accidents each the ratio of accidents among the members of B group over A became 5.09% to 1%.

Somewhat higher differences were obtained when the patients of the two groups were compared instead of their accidents.

The comparative frequency of multiple or repeated accidents in Groups A and B at different ages was first studied for the entire nineteen-year period: 1930 through 1948 and again as the sum total of four different periods: 1930-41, 1942-1944, 1945 and 1946-1948. The results obtained from both of these studies showed a high degree of correlation.

The higher incidence of accidents in the maladjusted and irresponsible families (Group B) was especially marked in the young patients under the age of twenty-five. Of all the multiple accidents in Group B, 85.2% occurred before the age of thirty-five and 71.5% before the age of twenty-five; while in Group A, only sixty per cent of the multiple accidents occurred before the age of thirty-five and only 44.5% before the age of twenty-five. Counting all the accidents, single as well as multiple, 79.2% of the accidents in Group B and 65.8% of those in Group A occurred before the age of thirty-five; while in females of Group B, nearly eighty-three per cent occurred during this period of time.

The difference in the accident frequency of the two groups was especially prominent in their children. The children of the maladjusted and irresponsible homes (Group B) were found to have a significantly higher incidence of accidents than the children of the normally adjusted families (Group A). In Group B, 30.7% of all the accidents occurred before the age of fifteen, while in Group A, only 21.6% of the accidents occurred before this age. The difference was even greater when the multiple or repeated accidents of the two groups were compared. In Group B, 46.2% of the multiple accidents occurred before the age of fifteen; while in Group A, only twenty-seven per cent occurred before the same age.

The difference in the frequency of accidents in these two groups of patients, according to age, were also highly significant. In Group A, the incidence of accidents decreased steadily from early childhood to the age of ten to fourteen, while in Group B, there was an increase in accident rate at the age of five to nine before the usual decline at the age of ten to fourteen. The contrast in the age distribution of patients with multiple or repeated accidents in Groups A and B was most remarkable. In Group A the incidence of multiple accidents remained at a relatively low and fairly even level of distribution, of eight to nine per cent, throughout the greater part of life or up to the age of fifty when they began to decrease with further increment in age. In Group B, on the other hand, multiple accidents rose precipitously to a high peak of twenty to twenty-one per cent at the young age of five to nine and then decreased steadily with increment in age. In Group A, the age distribution of the young patients with multiple accidents was only slightly above the normal age distribution of the general population of Cincinnati (U.S. Census, 1930 and 1940); while in Group B, the age distribution of the patients with multiple accidents under the age of twenty-five was significantly higher than either in Group A or in the general population.

In the total series of single and multiple accidents, the frequency rate increased slightly in boys at the age of five to nine; it then decreased at the age of ten to fourteen, rose to a peak at the age of twenty to twenty-four and then decreased steadily with increment in age. In the females of both groups and in all the patients of Group A, the same age distribution of accidents prevailed, except for lack of an increase in the frequency of accidents at the age of five to nine.

These studies indicate that persons belonging to maladjusted and irresponsible families tend to have a significantly higher incidence of accidents, solitary as well as multiple ones, than those not so designated. This group (B) is especially noted for the high rate of accidents among their children; particularly during the age of five to nine, an age when the over-all accident rate is otherwise low. At the usual peak age for accidents of twenty to twenty-four, the incidence in Group B was 16.4% compared to 14.1% in Group A.

From the foregoing it is apparent that a small percentage of a given population can account for most of the accidents on the basis of youth alone; or the presence in such a population of an undue number of irresponsible and maladjusted individuals. The presence of both of these factors at one and the same time would naturally accentuate the unequal distribution of the accidents.

An important group has thus been identified in the general population, the irresponsible and maladjusted group that has a high frequency of accidents or apparently contributes a disproportionate share to the total number of accidents. This high accident-frequency group has been further identified with regard to the ages at which most of the accidents occur. In contrast with other methods of study, the above described groups of "accident-prone" individuals are easily recognizable by means of a thorough clinical history.

It followed that an appreciable reduction in accident frequency may be expected through remedial steps consequent upon attention to maladjustment factors such as irresponsibility, insecurity, domestic strife, parent over-authority, anxiety and all those influences to be catalogued as the abnormal strains and conflicts of modern living.

CHAPTER NINE

HEALTH AND HANDICAPS

It is known that even a slight departure from good health may diminish muscular control and reduce the power of attention and concentration. Although an individual's deviation from normal good health may be insufficient to produce symptoms, it may be sufficient to increase his susceptibility to accidents. The precise relationship between health and accidents is not easy to measure or define. Two methods have been employed in studying this relationship: (a) comparing the number of accidents and the number of illnesses reported by each individual in a working group and, (b) comparing the number of accidents and the amount of time lost by each individual through illness.

Newbold (46) and Farmer and Chambers (20) found that the correlation between length of illness and accident frequency was insignificant. A British study (69) discloses that those who most often report sick with minor ailments in a working group have, on the whole, a higher accident rate than the others. Reports of other investigators have confirmed this observation. Like American investigators, the British have found no relationship between length of lost-time sickness and accident frequency. They propose, by way of explanation, that sickness rate expressed in terms of lost-time is a measure of the severity of illness and not of its incidence. They also suggest that the positive correlation between the number of minor illnesses and accidents may be due to a practice on the part of some individuals to report their sicknesses and accidents more often than others. The frequency with which minor ailments are reported is thus not necessarily a measure of the true incidence of illness or accidents in the group as a whole.

The tendency on the part of some individuals repeatedly to seek help for minor ailments or injuries may be an expression of the need for secondary psychological gain. However, it is well to bear in mind that some of those who report more frequently actually have a higher incidence of sickness and/or accidents than those who do not have this disposition. Conversely, the failure to seek medical aid does not in itself prove one way or another what the incidence of minor sickness and accidents is in these persons.

The lack of correlation between the amount of time lost as a result of illness and the number of accidents may be due in part to changes in the incidence and duration of illness or accidents which go with changes in age. After twenty-five years of age, as persons grow older, there is a steady decline in the incidence of accidents and an increase in the incidence of illness. The duration of illness also tends to increase with advancing years. In younger persons, on the other hand, both illness and accidents are often at peak levels of incidence, while the recovery periods are relatively short. Under these circumstances, one could hardly expect any marked degree of correlation between incidence of accidents and lost-time illness. Whatever the explanation, it seems clear on the face of the evidence, that the incidence of illness is related to accident rate and that the length of time lost by illness is not.

The British Industrial Health Research Board (69) suggests that measuring sickness rate by the number of times it is reported may introduce a better indication of general ill health than measuring it by the length of time lost as a result of it, since the frequent repetition of minor ailments may in itself be an indication of poor health. The same report suggests that the exertions and stresses of industrial life may put upon workers an undue strain and induce a state of nervousness which predisposes them to accidents.

Newbold (46) in 1926, investigated the records of a number of factories to determine the frequency of minor illness and accidents in six groups of men and women. The minor ailments consisted of headaches, colds, sore throats, indigestion, faintness, abdominal pains, toothaches, etc., and were all treated in the plant dispensary. Upon comparing the coefficient of correlation between the frequency of minor ailments and accidents, Newbold found that these ranged from

0.42 to 0.19 and averaged about 0.3. In other words, there was a low, though positive, correlation between the frequency of minor ailments and accidents.

Studying a group of three hundred and fifty-two metal workers, Newbold found that during a six-months period these men sustained one thousand three hundred and thirty accidents and that those who reported ill more frequently also reported more frequent accidents. Those who did not report sick during the six-months period averaged two accidents each; those who reported ill once or twice, had three or four accidents; those who reported ill three to five times, suffered about five accidents each, and those who reported ill eight to ten times, suffered about eight accidents each. By keeping the age and experience factors constant, it was found that the strong relationship between the frequency of minor illnesses and the frequency of accidents was not appreciably affected by the age and experience of the workers.

Vernon (60) reported several investigations which tend to show a positive correlation between hypertension or some of the conditions associated with it (especially nervousness) and high accident frequency. By a process of deductive reasoning, Vernon concluded that ". . . though evidence has not been obtained to show that the two groups are identical, it seems probable that they largely correspond."

Slocombe and Bingham (57, 62) studied the accident frequency and blood pressure readings of sixty-nine streetcar drivers over fifty years of age and found that while the thirty-eight men with normal blood pressure averaged three collision accidents, those with abnormal pressure averaged six and a half accidents. The other conditions associated with abnormal blood pressure were not reported.

Kirk (36A) studied a group of four hundred and twenty-two male industrial workers of all ages and found that thirty-six per cent had high blood pressure. The high blood pressure group also had a higher incidence of impaired vision, varicose veins and oral sepsis than the group of workers with normal blood pressure. Kirk also reported more obesity, a greater tendency for indulgence in alcoholic beverages and more nervousness and worrying in the high blood pressure group.

Soddy (58), in a study of the psychological aspects of accidents, declares that: "Accident-proneness is related to lack of quickness, slow reaction time, poor muscular coordination, poor intelligence, instability of temperament and distractibility." He suggests among other things that accidents should be studied as social events. "They occur as integral parts of our daily life in the community; we expect them and we should make provision for them."

According to Mauro (40), the human element is responsible for the majority of industrial accidents. In workers of either sex, the main causes of accidents include sight and hearing deficiencies, insufficient motor and reflex coordinations, alcoholism and fatigue. Industrial accidents are more frequent in young workers of either sex than in the older. In women, menstruation, pregnancy, lactation and menopause may have a predisposing role.

Murphy (45) attributes accidents to a great variety of causes. "Accidents and injuries seem to happen when apparently every known precaution has been put into effect to prevent their existence. Individual temperament, defects in eyesight or hearing, carelessness, improperly adjusted machinery, alcoholic intoxication, poor roads, inclement weather, improperly constructed building material, lack of attention, failure to obey orders, the thoughtlessness of youth and childhood, confusion in moments of stress or emergencies, are all factors which at times lead to accidents." . . . "Fear and rage each play a part in the production of accidents and injuries, for when reason is entirely overshadowed by such influences, responsibility is cast to the winds."

Culpin and Smith (15) reported an investigation of over a thousand men and women clerical and factory workers and students, using the interview method of study. They found that about twenty per cent of the subjects suffered from nervous symptoms which interfered with their happiness and efficiency. This group also gave poor results with the McDougall-Schuster dotting test. Farmer and Chamber (20) similarly found that twenty per cent of the workers tested by them had a higher incidence of accidents and tended to do the dotting test badly. The possible correlation between these two conditions has not been determined.

Culpin (16) reported a study of one thousand five hundred persons whom he examined at work, with the aim of estimating the prevalence of psychoneurotic symptoms in people who reach the physician in search of relief. He found that from five to seven per cent of the working population suffer to that extent. About twenty per cent have lesser symptoms to interfere with efficiency and happiness, twenty per cent present an odd symptom or so that does not affect them, while forty to fifty per cent reveal no symptoms on superficial examination.

Although the statistical evidence seems to be rather tenuous, it appears probable that the twenty to thirty per cent of the population who suffer from neurotic symptoms at any given time are, in large part, the same twenty to thirty per cent of the population who have most of the accidents at any given time of study. Only a relatively small percentage of those who present symptoms of neurosis and those with a high accident frequency are relatively fixed in their neurotic behavior and/or accident habit. Almost any person may respond with neurotic symptoms and/or accidents under the stimulus of appropriate stressful life situations.

This point of view is supported by Vernon (60) who concluded that "the accident-proneness of various individuals is not a fixed quality, but is liable to be affected by any and every change in the bodily condition. This condition is influenced by external changes of environment as well as by internal changes of physical and mental health."

Bills (11), in 1931, reported a relationship between "mental fatigue" and errors which may possibly have a bearing on some accidents. After extensive experimentation, Bills found that "in mental work involving considerable homogeneity and continuity, there occur, with almost rhythmic regularity, blocks or pauses during which no response occurs." The "blocks" or pauses occur at an average rate of about three per minute; they tend to decrease in frequency and size with practice and to increase with fatigue. The tendency for errors to occur in conjunction with "blocks" suggests that the cause of errors lies in recurrent states of low mental functioning which the "blocks" reveal.

Larson et al. (38A), in a recent publication, reviewed some one hundred psychological and sociological studies of industrial accidents. Their conclusions may be summarized as follows:

1. Most industrial accidents can be attributed to human behavior.

2. The importance of such factors as reaction time, manual dexterity, and visual abilities in accident causation varies with the

type of activity. Of greater importance are such factors as anticipation, atention, proper lighting, fatigue and a general predisposition to work in a safe manner.

3. Tests for intelligence, general coordination, hand-finger skill, arm-hand facility and knowledge of mechanical operations do not identify accident-free workers from accident repeaters except at the extremes. These tests are of some help where exceptional abilities are essential to safe performance. To a certain extent an interest in mechanical things seems to be associated with safe workers.

4. Personality has a great deal to do with accidents. Of special importance are the degree of adjustment of the individual to everyday living and his ability to get along with others.

5. Physically impaired workers who have adjusted psychologically and vocationally to their limitations are good safety risks.

6. The degree of adjustment of a new employee to his new work setting is an important indication of his future work and accident record.

7. Well-trained employees usually have fewer accidents than poorly trained or maltrained workers.

8. Attention to machinery design, machine guards, plant layouts, lighting facilities, paint color, and house cleaning activities, have consistently benefited accident experience. Yet accidents continue to occur after all of these have been included in plant operations.

9. Peak accident hours generally coincide with peak fatigue hours. Ways of counteracting the effects of fatigue include sound proofing, carefully planned music programs, five-meal eating schedules and periodic well-timed rest periods.

10. Accidents increase with decrease in employee morale.

11. Accidents will continue to occur even with ideal hiring procedures, proper training programs, good supervision, ideal physical working conditions, good morale and a generally satisfied work force. Further improvement in accident experience may be achieved through certain detailed information about each individual worker and a reliable history of his past behavior and accidents.

PHYSICAL HANDICAPS

Orthopedically handicapped persons do not, as a rule, meet with accidents more often than those not so afflicted. The handicapped person is instinctively more careful and more alert to danger. This does not apply to physically handicapped children and older disabled persons who may require special care and attention to safeguard them from accidents. The above is the prevailing view in the literature, and is contrary to an earlier opinion based largely on investigations by Viteles (63), interpreted to mean that men with physical defects have more accidents than those without.

Viteles studied the relationship between physical defects and accident frequency in a group of one hundred and six electrical substation operators. These were divided into two main groups: (a) fifty-seven men without physical defects, and (b) thirty-one men with some physical defect plus eighteen other men who for various reasons were not considered fit for their position. An analysis of the lost-time accidents of these two groups of employees over a ten-year period showed that the average time lost by the physically handicapped was three times greater than by those without defects. The average age of group (b) was 38.5 or six years older than group (a); while the length of service was three years longer.

This study of Viteles may be criticized on several grounds: (1) Group (b) was a mixed group consisting two-thirds of physically handicapped and one-third of rejectees. The latter sub-group may have included emotionally unstable, maladjusted and irresponsible individuals or individuals with a high accident potential due to personality defect. Most observers would agree that the inclusion in group (b) of persons without physical defects greatly weakens the conclusions drawn from this study. (2) The greater loss of time following injury in group (b) may have been related to the physical and other incapacities of the group rather than to increased "accident liability." Again, the loss of time following injury is a measure of the severity rather than the frequency of accidents. (3) The longer convalescence in group (b) was, of course, partly due to the slower recuperative power of this older age group.

Aisenson (5) reviewed the records of nine hundred and sixty resident patients engaged in a full athletic program at a children's psychiatric hospital in order to compare the incidence of potentially serious injuries in convulsive and non-convulsive children. Of two hundred and ten convulsive children, 2.8% were so injured, while of seven hundred and fifty non-convulsive children, 2.9% were so injured. Since no extra risk of injury was found in the convulsive children, the author proposed that they be allowed full participation on physical education programs in schools and camps.

Miller and Ross (44) reported a most unusual study. These authors found that the aortic size in accident cases is significantly smaller than in patients dying of ordinary hospital diseases. They found that the degree of scatter of sizes (measured by the variance) is significantly smaller in the accident group. Measurements were taken of the circumference of three hundred aortas and studied in relation to age, body weight, height and sex. The mean size, only corrected for these four variates in patients dying from accident, was significantly smaller than those dying from disease.

According to the authors, two alternative explanations are available: first, that there is some causal connection between the aortic size and the chance of death by accident; or secondly, that people dying from ordinary hospital diseases have aortas dilated above the normal size by some causal factor unconnected with age, weight, height or sex, while the accident cases have normal aortas.

Miller and Ross conclude: "While the choice between the alternatives remains open, it seems more likely that the first is correct—that there is a more or less well defined group of people with narrow aortas who are specially liable to accidental death. It is difficult to believe that the connection is a direct one. An indirect connection seems more likely. Arterial hypoplasia is a leading feature in so-called 'status lymphaticus' and here the condition is a developmental one. There is also frequently some degree of feminine habitus in the male. The general impression is that 'status lymphaticus' cases have a poor resistance to infection, but the absence of a suitable criterion as to what constitutes good or poor resistance precludes the addition of such cases to the figures for accidental deaths."

MOOD SWINGS

Hersey (34) made an extensive study of the moods and emotional experiences of a group of industrial workers of varied ages. The author was primarily interested in mood swings or cycles as they affected fatigability and efficiency.

Hersey began his study with twenty-seven persons selected for varying temperaments and habits and ranging in age from eighteen to sixty-three years. For nearly two years, he practically lived with the group. He interviewed each of them twice and most of them four times daily. At each interview the exact state of their feelings and how the world looked to them was talked over carefully and charted on the scale. Every circumstance that might seem to cause the person's then-present emotions was considered. Each man tried to answer as accurately as possible as to his sleep, digestion, mood, worry, losses, sense of humor, effect of jokes, his exact sex relations in the past twenty-four hours, consumption of alcohol, coffee or tobacco, etc. Every circumstance that might affect the man's emotions temporarily or permanently was discussed with absolute frankness. Detailed physical examinations and laboratory studies of these individuals were made periodically to determine the existence of any possible relationship between the emotional and physical states of the individual.

Hersey concluded that at certain predictable periods there is a lowering of one's emotional resistance to the stresses of life and that these ebbs in mood are usually marked by a lessening of physical energy and self-control. During these periods of depression, it is not only more difficult to deal with problems and disappointments, but even favorable news fails to have a "lifting" effect. Hersey noted that happiness runs in cycles and that circumstances have little to do with determining the depressions. Each person swings up out of his "low" into a rather characteristic zone in which he remains for several weeks, with short minor ups and downs. The troughs on the low side usually begin and end rather suddenly and last from four to six days. In young persons under the age of twenty, the cycle runs only approximately fourteen to sixteen days, with but a day and a half or two days in the trough.

Although the "highs" are all pretty much alike, there are three different types of "lows." In the first of these three types of "lows," productive powers are about ten per cent below normal and the subject is depressed but not desperate. With extra effort he can produce the normal amount; about sixty per cent of all "lows" are of this type. In a second type, neither drink, self-chiding nor love can pull him up to normal. It is at such times that people attempt suicide; this type covers about one-fourth of the "lows." In the third type of "low" the man is depressed mentally, but his physical energy is high and often he cannot control it. This type explains many boxing and sports upsets and covers about fifteen per cent of the "lows."

According to Hersey there seems to be a distinct relationship between the happiness cycle and the sex urge and activities in men, but not in women. In married men, the sex urge is keenest at both the highest and lowest points of the cycle. In unmarried men, the sex urge is very mild or absent during the low period. In women, there seems to be no relationship between the emotional and menstrual cycle. It seems strongly indicated that if a woman is in the high portion of her happiness cycle at the menstrual period, she suffers little or no depression. If she is in the low part of her happiness cycle during her menstrual period, she suffers profound depression.

Hersey feels that mood swings or happiness cycles offer a new approach to the understanding of accidents, fatigue, mental and bodily efficiency, sense of humor, drinking, smoking and the like. Hersey's study has been severely criticized on methodological grounds, yet there seems to be some validity to his main conclusions on the basis of everyday experience.

Benedek and Rubenstein (9) investigated the correlation between the gonad cycle and the emotional cycle. Vaginal smear and basal body temperature techniques were used as means of assaying endocrinological states and psychoanalysis was applied for predicting the hormonal state. The subjects were fifteen women of childbearing age and one hundred fifty-two cycles were collected on each. Preliminary conclusions drawn from seventy-five cycles of nine patients indicated "a correlation between each hormonal variation of the sexual cycle and the psychodynamic manifestations of the sexual drive." The authors state that definite relationship exists between hormone cycles and psychosexual development, justfying the view that the sexual cycle is a psychosomatic unit.

McCance *et al.* (41) investigated physical and emotional periodicity in women. They collected records over a period of four to six months of one hundred sixty-seven normal women's physical changes and subjective phenomena. The results indicated that many physical and mental symptoms in women are in some cases unexpectedly rhythmical. The authors list these symptoms in their order of frequency as follows: fatigue, depression, breast changes, headache, abdominal pain and backache. They found some association between fatigue and depression. Elation and depression, however, were not found to be complementary in distribution.

Billings (10), in 1934, investigated the cycle variations in motor activity in relation to the menstrual cycle in the human female. A pedometer was used as the instrument of measurement. The amount of estrogenic substance in the blood was determined once weekly by the biological test of Frank. This study indicated: (1) that there is a time relationship between secretions of hormones and activity which is synchronous with phases of the menstrual cycle; (2) that there is a suggested correlation between the degree of motor activity and the amount of estrogenic substance in the blood; (3) that without overt signs of menstruation, there are certain fairly regular ovarian-function cycles, and (4) that these cycles are made more regular, more pronounced and gradually return more nearly to normal following the administration of thyroid extract.

All considered, it does not appear to be established that an acceptable correlation may be located between accident rates and the frequency of organic diseases. Undoubtedly there are exceptions with respect to individual diseases possibly including hyperthyroidism. As to functional disorders and with particular reference to functional mental disorders, the situation is different, but that consideration reaches into the domain of maladjustment, anxiety, etc., not contemplated in this chapter.

CHAPTER TEN

THE CLINICAL MEDICAL APPROACH

THE hope is that the contents of this text will have engendered the over-all conclusion that future major gains in the prevention of eighty-five per cent of all accidents devolve upon the medical profession. Past major gains were achieved by all those measures commonly catalogued as "safety" and through training and education. Those media have earned unstinted acclaim, but have exhausted their possibilities as to added accomplishments anywhere near their early successes. There is utterly no disposition to minimize these contributions. All such efforts must be continued and even enlarged, but the most that may be expected is the maintenance of what already has been reached.

There exists no innovation in the assertion that future large scale returns from efforts directed toward accident prevention depend upon activities of the medical profession. That conclusion has been reached by a host of investigators. What is new is the realization that for foreseeable time this is the only approach of promise. The human mind, warped in mild fashion or grossly, is the area of opportunity and only the skilled may enter.

A diagnosis has been made. A diagnosis alone is not sufficient. As in much of medicine, a precise diagnosis may afford scientific satisfaction, but not always does it provide remedy and betimes remedy is never attainable. As to human minds and accident causation, there remains after the diagnosis the need to scrutinize and appraise what and how betterment may be attained.

The difficulties are gigantic. The number of needy minds is to be counted in myriads. No brain, however to be labeled as stable, escapes all lapses. These mild and temporary deviations frequently are the source of accidents, but such fleeting mental quirks do not demand the immediate ministrations of psychiatrists. Laying aside those millions who through self-discipline and analysis right their own maladjustments, there remains that uncounted throng among whom maladjustment is the rule, either continuous or continual. Any attempt to provide numbers invites unfavorable criticism of speculation, but there are those who assert that some seventy per cent of the adult population engage in practices and activities that warrant the label of "poor judgment," "juvenility" or the like. Whatever be the number or percentages, never is it a fixed group. Always recruitment and escape is going on. Whatever be the number and how permanent or temporary be their state of mental maladjustment—these are the accident-makers.

The human mind is not something to be meddled with under the guise of psychotherapy. It may be promptly recorded that the average good physician lacks qualification to invade the mind beyond surface levels and rarely does he consider himself adequate to meet psychiatric needs. The practitioner of general medicine may serve well indeed by making a working diagnosis and by treating the vast majority of these patients through establishing rapport, extending sympathy when justified and fulfilling obvious needs for human relationship and understanding; beyond that, he may serve best through reliance upon the superior skill of the functional psychiatrist.

Now having attempted to set limits for the physician, less complaint will arise if this same negation is directed to other groups. Fully and for all time the pseudo-psychologists are to be condemned. They constitute a malignant and pestiferous menace. Unfortunately they may possess the appeal of glibness far above that of the skilled psychologist whom they presume to ape. Should there be a determination to utilize the services of an industrial psychologist, how may management determine qualifications? In the first place, the genuine psychologist never conducts mass meetings after lurid advertising nor does he peddle his wares in blandishments spread out on the manager's desk. When in doubt, one may consult any local medical society, any established and respected psychiatrist or any industrial medical director.

Probing the human mind is not for mass action. The traits of human frailties and failings are peculiarly individualistic. But it is reckless to assert that nothing is to be won by mass approaches. Many persons are buoyed by suitable morale building or inspirational presentations. For example, let it be assumed that a mass meeting is centered about "speed." Clearly excessive speed is a threat to automobile travel and to industrial work. Truly, speed often is the revealment of the workings of at least a score of those two hundred fifty and more factors that contribute to mental maladjustment. Such a mass meeting on "speed" may accomplish much and perhaps chiefly on the basis of joint response, the individual responder not wanting to be apart from the group. Still, any result will fail signally in uprooting from the individual his particular background of causation that provoked the recklessness of which speed is but one manifestation.

Assembled groups of parents afford some opportunity for fending the ravages of mental distortion in their children. If all parents were the best of parents, and long had been, this book probably never would have been written. But who will say what is "best?" Were there no delinquent parents, there would be few delinquent children.

The safety engineer and those who serve in safety without being graduate engineers, in industry and elsewhere, have both particular opportunities and sharp limitations in this approach to accident reduction by way of the disturbed mind. Without debate the safety engineer in his training role should not assay the fundamental role of the psychiatrist or psychologist, but well he may function on the fringes. A pleasant slap on the back at the right moment sometimes may be more valuable psychologically than two years of deep pervasion of the mind by the psychoanalyst. Confronted with a recalcitrant workman who refuses to wear protective goggles in a dangerous area, the perplexed safety engineer may not realize that the resistance unconsciously is directed to the department foreman who has become the surrogate father of the belligerent workman, who thus transfers his hostility for his own father. Even if the engineer were aware of these mental cross wires, he is not the one to do the uncrossing. Were the workman transferred to another department, the hostility likely would be implanted elsewhere.

On the positive and constructive side, all is not hopeless.

In industry skilled, specially trained nurses often are successful in psychological counseling.

A demanding need is for the training of all medical students better to function as psychiatrically oriented physicians whether in general practice or in the specialties. In all of medical practice, there are continuing opportunities for the application of judicious psychotherapy but for any such to have helpful meaning there must have been prior training to competency in sound psychiatry even though the level be well below that of the specialized psychiatrist.

Perhaps no fewer than ten thousand additional professional psychiatrists and psychologists are needed to take over the confirmed "accident-repeaters" extensively described in this book.

More and more the law enforcing agencies would do well to do more than punish. Judicious punishment may be salutary, but it removes few mental maladjustments and may make more. The court psychiatrist deserves a freer hand, and is it beyond reasonableness that a few judges be psychiatrists?

Indisputably the grade school teacher becomes a member of this mental maladjustment removal team. Neglectful parents, and thus nearly all parents, impose upon school teachers all too much of normal parental responsibility. This responsibility is being accepted and so being, teachers need every iota of proper qualifications suited to the making non-operative those scores of factors conducive to lifetime accident causation.

A prime attainment at the present time would seem to be a unified, intensive, basic research program by teams of clinicians and other workers in the related sciences. There is a profitable occasion for an educational program aimed at a broader understanding of the nature of the problem and a more hopeful outlook. It should be stressed that an accident is basically an avoidable morbid condition and that an accident-patient may be in need of therapeutic or preventive medical aid aside from the care of his injuries. For maximum effectiveness, physicians should learn to recognize the dynamic forces that play a role in accident causation and learn to recognize and treat the accident syndrome.

Unless vigorous application of the approach here proposed be espoused, or others of equal or greater promise if there be such, then the present appalling accident frequency will continue. In the United States in 1953 one of every sixteen persons incurred a disabling injury. For every disabling injury more than one hundred lesser accidents arose. All are important.

CHAPTER ELEVEN

SUMMATION* (53)

Accidents are an age-old problem, and their prevention was already a matter of serious concern in early Biblical times. Since the turn of the present century, accidents have been studied most intensively. Yet, despite four decades of heroic preventive efforts and some notable achievements, the accident toll remains staggeringly high. The annual cost of accidents in the U.S.A. has remained for many years at approximately one hundred thousand killed, four hundred thousand permanently disabled, ten million injured, with one or more days of disability, and ten billion dollars of direct and indirect expenditures. There is a serious accident in every fifth household annually, and every single day of the week an average of two hundred sixty persons are killed and twenty-six thousand are injured.

The accident problem looms even bigger in face of the large percentage of young persons, in their prime of life, who are injured, killed or crippled by accidents. The anxiety, the pain, the mental anguish stirred up and the emotional disequilibrium into which many family groups are thrown as a result of accidents and their social and economic concomitants are also important. Considering the seriousness of the problem and the progress which has been made in reducing morbidity and mortality from other causes, the meager amount of basic research being reported on the subject of accidents is another cause for concern.

The author's interest in accidents dates back to the year 1930 when he entered the industrial and general practice of medicine. By choice and from the beginning the major part of his practice was devoted

---

*From a paper read before the Section on Preventive and Industrial Medicine and Public Health at the 103rd Annual Meeting of the American Medical Association, San Francisco, June 22, 1954.

to the care of the injured. Since the accident problem is still an open one, a study of accumulated case histories was undertaken in 1947 which eventually included thirty-eight thousand cases. These represented twenty-seven thousand industrial accidents, eight thousand non-industrial accidents and three thousand cases of illness from all causes, studied for the purpose of comparison.

This group of patients differs in many respects from those studied by others. It was not limited to industrial accidents, or to one or a few plants, industries, occupations, age groups, or types of injury. The accidents occurred in the home, at work, in public places, in schools, and on the road. The patients were of all social, economic and cultural levels and represented nearly all occupations and industries, most of the plants, and many of the business establishments of a large mid-western community.

The investigations yielded new facts as well as confirmations and refutations of some old theories. The studies suggest that the widely accepted theory attributing most accidents to a "small fixed group of 'accident-prone' individuals who cannot help from having accidents" is open to question. They indicate, instead, that when the period of observation is sufficiently long, the "small group of individuals who are responsible for most of the accidents" is essentially a changing group, with new persons constantly falling in and out of the group (55). Accidents appear to be a wide-spread endemic affliction, and seem to be part of a disease syndrome—the accident syndrome. Most accidents were observed to conform to a pattern, having a known though varied etiology, distinctive prodromal signs, symptoms and circumstances and are thus frequently predictable.

The more important and pertinent findings which have led to the foregoing conclusions may be summarized as follows:

1. Accidents are essentially an affliction of youth, decreasing steadily after reaching a peak at the age of twenty-one.

2. Males have a significantly higher incidence of accidents than females (2:1). This is true for every single year of the normal life span, except the first, and in every type of activity, except the handling of household objects.

3. Most accidents (seventy-four per cent) are due to relatively infrequent solitary experiences of large numbers of individuals (eighty-

six per cent). These percentages were identical in industrial as well as in non-industrial accidents, and remained constant nearly every year of a twenty-year period.

4. Irresponsible and maladjusted individuals have a significantly higher incidence of accidents, especially repeated ones, than responsible and normally adjusted individuals.

5. The incidence of accidents follows a relatively fixed annual cyclical pattern of distribution, increasing steadily from a low in February to a high in June and August and then decreasing steadily to the low.

6. The incidence of non-industrial accidents follows a relatively fixed diurnal cyclical pattern of distribution, increasing steadily from a low at 5:00 a. m. to a peak at 5:00 p.m., and then decreasing again.

7. Eighty per cent of non-industrial accidents belong to one of six types: Falls, aggressive behavior, handling objects, foreign bodies, motor vehicles and stumbling into objects.

8. Accidents often occur in chain fashion as if one accident acted as a trigger mechanism or as a sensitising agent, for another accident or series of accidents in the individual or the group.

9. In about fifty per cent of those having repeated accidents (3+) they occur during identical hours. This tendency increases with the number of accidents per patient.

10. Some persons tend to repeat accidents on certain days of the week or month, particularly on days with special significance to the individual.

11. There are those who have a predilection for certain types of accident or for injury to certain parts of the body.

12. In all types of individuals, accidents are more likely to occur under the influence of emotional stress or strain.

The last group of observations (8-12) tends to support the findings of others that psychological factors play a role in the genesis of some accidents, and that some accidents and injuries may have symbolic significance to the individual. No adequate statistical studies are available, as yet, to indicate the relative importance of these factors.

With the aid of the foregoing findings and parts of the literature, the writer proposes that it is now possible to predict with reasonable certainty when, to whom, under what conditions and in what circumstances, an accident is most likely and least likely to occur. An accident is *most* likely to occur to: a young man, age twenty-one; on a hot and humid summer day; during the months of June and July; on a week-end or a holiday; while driving a car or with aggressive behavior; during the late evening hours if not working; or during the homeward rush hours of the late afternoon and early evening, especially if these are also the hours of darkness.

The likelihood of an accident increases further with inexperience; with excessive speed; the partaking of alcoholic beverages; physiological or psychological fatigue; with certain specific psychological conflicts; and with the degree or intensity of such non-specific emotional factors as anxiety, hostility, frustration, and guilt. The chances for an accident are greatest if the young man is irresponsible and maladjusted; grew up in a maladjusted home; and was exposed in childhood to violence and strife, to over-authoritative parents or parent figures, to separation or loss of parents, and to accidents to himself, parents or siblings. The probability of an accident also grows with any increase in the duration or intensity of exposure to environmental hazards.

An accident is *least* likely to occur in a healthy well-adjusted young girl, age thirteen, born and reared in a normal, secure and loving home, in which both parents are well adjusted and if she has not experienced or witnessed major or frequent accidents in the past. The likelihood of an accident decreases further with the hours of night, the month of February, the mid-week, the home environment and a minimal exposure to hazards. Even with increased exposure and increased physical, physiological or psychological stress or strain, an accident is relatively unlikely to occur in this type of individual.

Between these extremes there are an endless number of possible combinations of factors, capable of yielding varying degrees of accident probability. A working familiarity with the more important accident factors and the prevailing combinations of factors should enable the clinician to evaluate the probability of an accident in any given set of circumstances or individuals.

Of the more than two hundred and fifty accident factors mentioned in the literature, many are of minor or doubtful importance and few have been studied exhaustively or conclusively. Research leading to the pin-pointing or quantitating of at least the more important accident factors should be of great help to the physician in the diagnosis, prevention and treatment of the accident syndrome. The ability to diagnose this syndrome depends on an intimate knowledge of predisposing factors, environmental hazards, known trigger mechanisms and a past history of the behavior pattern of the individual when confronted with a sudden decision or danger.

From the findings presented earlier, it can be computed that, on the basis of age and sex distribution alone, a small percentage of a given population could account for most of the accidents. Pure chance is, of course, also a factor in the unequal distribution of accidents. The presence of an undue number of highly "accident-prone" individuals would naturally accentuate the unequal distribution of accidents due to age, sex and chance. Our studies suggest that, when the period of observation is sufficiently long, most accidents occur in individuals with a low degree of proneness, and that the relatively small percentage of the population that contributes a disproportionate number of accidents is essentially a shifting group, with new persons constantly falling in and out of the group.

In the course of a lifetime almost any normal individual under emotional stress may become temporarily "accident-prone" and may suffer a series of accidents in fairly rapid succession. Most persons, however, find solutions to their problems, develop defenses against their emotional conflicts, and drop out of the highly "accident-prone" group after a few hours, days, weeks or months. Some individuals may remain highly "accident-prone" throughout life, with or without lapses of years of freedom from the accident habit. The latter are the truly "accident-prone" individuals. They contribute, however, only a relatively small percentage of all the accidents.

On the basis of experience and the evidence presented, accidents appear to be a widespread endemic affliction affecting most individuals many times in the course of a lifetime. The excessive liability to accidents in youth usually disappears with age and in most accident repeaters, with learning, with physiological and psychological adaptation, with the development of more adequate psychological defenses, the elimination of hazardous exposure, etc.

If we were to pin-point the main groups of "accident-makers" they would be found among the young, the male and the maladjusted; with unbridled, misdirected aggressiveness a uniting common denominator. Repeated accidents are most frequently encountered in the above three groups, while "true" or "fixed" "accident-proneness" is a rarity. For more than two decades now, a tremendous effort has gone into the finding, re-educating, eliminating or rendering harmless the "small group of individuals who cause most of the accidents"—the "accident-prones." Although studies of "accident-proneness" have been fascinating and instructive, they have often resulted in a fruitless chase of a phantom group. Greater promise towards accident reduction, beyond the presently successful efforts in "safety," seems to lie in the direction of the clinical approach.

Viewing accidents as a disease syndrome has the advantage of focusing attention on this serious and widespread condition as a clinical entity, not merely as a problem in "safety." It may serve to reorient physicians to a consideration of the causes, prevention and clinical treatment of accidents per se, instead of the almost exclusive preoccupation with only one of the sequelae or surface manifestations of accidents—the injury. While emphasizing the importance of personality and of temporal factors in accident causation, the present theory can readily accommodate all other accident-producing and accident-predisposing factors. It has the added advantage of replacing the essentially fatalistic concept of "accident-proneness" by a more hopeful theory of accident causation.

The accident syndrome may be defined as a dynamic variable constellation of signs, symptoms and circumstances which together determine or influence the occurrence of an accident. This syndrome represents a synthesis of environmental, psychological, physiological, characterologic and temporal factors to form a unified theory of accident causation. The accident syndrome may also be described schematically as a morbid condition in which the elements of: (1) universal risk, (2) abnormal environment; (3) maladjustment and irresponsibility; (4) a trigger episode, and (5) behavior in the presence of the trigger episode combine to determine or influence the occurrence of the accident *(Frontispiece)*.

The component parts of the accident syndrome are not always well delineated. "Universal risk," in the main, represents the ever-present dangers, especially those in nature, the elements and chance, while "abnormal physical environment" largely includes man-made hazards. The dangers inherent in "universal risk" are usually of equal liability, while those related to "abnormal physical environment" are frequently selective, on the basis of occupation or type of activity.

All persons are subject to universal risks, especially to such natural forces as wind, snow, heat, ice, water, gravity, etc. The likelihood of an accident increases when there are abnormal environmental conditions. Here, the man-made hazards are of primary importance as for example, vehicles, machinery, fire, electricity, toxic substances, etc.

Accident liability is still more enhanced when the individual is irresponsible or maladjusted. These traits may be temporary or prolonged and may manifest themselves by flightiness, quickness to anger, absent-mindedness, carelessness, arrogance, defensiveness, frequent changes in residence or occupation, etc.

There is a trigger episode in every accident, usually referred to as the "cause" of the accident. The trigger may be a fleeting loss of balance, a rash decision, a miscalculated act, a driver doing the wrong thing, or whatever can precipitate the mishap. The trigger incident, which sets off the accident, may be part of the abnormal environment or of the human element. The trigger may be distinguished by its accelerated dynamics and by its intimate relationship to the final phase of the accident.

Human behavior in the presence of the trigger is often the final determinant in the occurrence and the character of the accident. The pattern of behavior of the individual, when confronted with a sudden decision or danger, will frequently determine whether the forces set in motion will result in a near-miss or in an accident.

Some may prefer to view accident causation in terms of the well known epidemiological triad of environment, host, and agent. In this representation, "universal risk" and "abnormal physical environment" would parallel the environmental factor; physical defects, mental maladjustment and behavior would equate the human or host factor, while the trigger episode would represent the agent.

Regardless of dynamics or theories of causation, it is evident that the cruel and clock-like regularity with which, year after year, many thousands of persons are killed, crippled and injured as a result of accidents, decidedly places this condition in the category of an endemic affliction of major proportions. It appears to the writer that the challenge which the accident problem presents should be met by a new and a more aggressive approach, directed primarily at the individual. Foremost is the need for an intensive, basic research program by teams of clinicians and other workers in the related sciences. There is also need for an educational program aimed at a wider general awareness of the full scope of the menace, a broader understanding of the nature of the problem and a more hopeful outlook. It should be stressed that an accident is basically an avoidable morbid condition; that any accident may result in tragedy or death; and that an accident-patient may be in need of therapeutic or preventive medical aid aside from the care of his injuries.

All available educational facilities, including mass media, should be utilized in a carefully conceived ceaseless educational effort. It seems highly improbable that accidents could be ballyhooed or legislated out of existence any more than could poliomyelitis, cancer, alcoholism or mental illness. Such methods are largely born of desperation and are grounded in the long lingering, hard-to-die notion that accidents are limited to a small, permanently stigmatized group of individuals, or more specifically, that they are due to "the carelessness, stupidity, ignorance, incompetence, irresponsibility or 'accident-proneness' of a small segment of the population." To be sure, all of these elements may be well represented in any large group, but the problem is not limited to these types of individuals and the implicated factors are usually too complex to be resolved by mere threats of punishment or disapprobation.

Accident prevention programs in industry have demonstrated that successful efforts depend on three essentials: (1) Rigid control of hazards, (2) Fitting the man into the job, and (3) Adequate motivation. It immediately becomes apparent that in a democracy such measures cannot be employed successfully, except with the active approval and cooperation of an enlightened public opinion. In accidents, as in other human ills, basic and lasting enlightenment must begin in the home and be continued in the schools. In industry a unique opportunity exists for effective adult education. In our stress ridden society, the very lives of countless thousands of individuals may literally depend on the effectiveness of such efforts.

In the light of the evidence, it would seem that educational and preventive programs must include the entire population since ultimately it is all of the population that is involved in all of the accidents. At the same time, it may be well to remember that individuals do vary in their susceptibility to accidents, as a result of certain childhood experiences and with age, sex, season, time of day, personality, mental and physical states, types of activity, special hazards, etc. Accident prevention must, therefore, concern itself with the individual as well as the group, with universal phenomena as well as with factors which are only of limited or local importance. It may be considered axiomatic that no one is immune to accidents and that even a trivial factor can be of utmost importance in the causation of some mishap.

Many are the skills that have affected accident experience favorably in the past and all of these should be utilized in the future. Yet, in the final analysis, accidents are a medical problem, and further major improvements in accident prevention must be in terms of clinical medicine with special emphasis on the adjustment of the individual to himself and to his environment. It follows that the foremost role in accident prevention should be relegated to the physician and to the time-honored doctor-patient relationship. In accidents, as in other forms of human morbidity, physicians should be on the alert for stressful life situations and they should utilize their special skills to relieve associated anxiety by appropriate means. For maximum effectiveness, physicians should learn to recognize the factors or forces which play a role in accident causation and they should learn to diagnose and treat the accident syndrome.

BIBLIOGRAPHY

1. ACKERMAN, N. W. AND CHIDESTER, L.: "Accidental" self-injury in children, *Arch. Pediat.*, *53*:711-721 (Nov.) 1936.
2. ADELSTEIN, A. M.: Unpublished doctoral dissertation on the accident rates of railway operatives, Univ. of the Witwatersrand, South Africa, 1951. *Ibid.*, Arbous (6).
3. ADLER, A.: Effect of trauma on psychological reactions, Wien. med. Wchnschr. 84: 293-295 (March 10) 1934.
4. ———: Psychology of repeated accidents, *Am. J. Psychiat.*, *98*:99-101 (July) 1941.
5. AISENSON, M. R.: Accidental injuries to epileptic children, *J. Pediat.*, *2*:85-88 (July) 1948.
6. ALEXANDER, FRANZ: The accident-prone individual, *Current Topics in Home Safety*, Vol. 32, 1948.
7. ARBOUS, A. G. AND KERRICH, J. D.: Accident statistics and the concept of accident proneness. Nat. Inst. for Personnel Res., South African Counc. for Scient. & Ind. Res. *Biometrics*, *7:*4, 1951. The phenomenon of accident proneness. *Indust. Med. & Surg.*, *22*:141-148 (April) 1953.
8. BAKWIN, R. M. AND H.: Accident proneness. *J. Pediat.*, *32*:749-752 (June) 1948.
9. BENEDEK, T. AND RUBENSTEIN, B. B.: The gonad cycle and the emotional cycle. *Rev. psicoanal.*, *1*:247-266 (Oct.) 1943.
10. BILLINGS, E. G.: The occurrence of cyclic variations in motor activity in relation to the menstrual cycle in the human female. *Bull. Johns Hopkins Hosp.*, *54*:440, 1934.
11. BILLS, A. G.: Blocking, a new principle of mental fatigue. *Am. J. Psychol.*, *43*:230, 1931.
12. BOND, DOUGLAS D.: *The Love and Fear of Flying.* New York, Internat. Univ. Press, 1952.
13. CHAMBERS, N. D. AND REISER, M. F.: Emotional stress in the precipitation of congestive heart failure. *Psychosom. Med.*, *15*:38-60 (Jan.-Feb.) 1953.
14. CSILLAG, I. AND HEDRI, E., JR.: Personal factors of accident proneness. *Indust. Med.*, *18*:29-30 (Jan.) 1949.
15. CULPIN, M. AND SMITH, M.: The nervous temperament. Indust. Health Research Board, Rep. No. 61, 1930.

16. ———: Psychological disorders in industry. *Practitioner, 137*:324-333, 1936.
17. DUNBAR, F.: *Psychosomatic Diagnosis.* New York & London, Paul B. Hoeber, Inc., Med. Book Dept. of Harper & Bros., 1943.
18. DUNBAR, FLANDERS, *et al*: Psychiatric aspects of medical problems. The psychic component of the disease process (including convalescence) in cardiac, diabetic and fracture patients. *Am. J. Psych., Part I, 93*:649-579 (November) 1936; Part II, *95*:1319-1342 (May) 1939.
19. FABIAN, A. A. AND BENDER, L.: Head injury in children. *Am. J. Orthopsychiat., 17*:68-79, 1947.
20. FARMER, E. AND CHAMBERS, E. G.: A psychological study of individual differences in accident rates, Indust. Health Research Board. Rep. No. 38, H. M. Stat. Office, 1926.
21. ——— AND CHAMBERS, E. G.: A study of accident proneness among motor drivers. Indust. Health Research Board, Rep. No. 84, 1939.
22. FETTERMAN, J. L.: *The Mind of the Injured Man.* Chicago, Indust. Med. Book Co., 1943.
23. ———: Aspects of industrial accidents. *Indust. Med., 15*:96-100 (Feb.) 1946.
24. FORSTER, N. K.: Mental attitudes. *Indust. Med., 6*:193-195 (April) 1937.
25. FREUD, S.: *Gesammelte Schriften,* Bd., I-XII, Leipzig, Internat. Psychoanalyt. Verlag, 1925.
26. ———: Psychopathology of everyday life. *Basic Writings of Sigmund Freud,* New York, Modern Library, 1938.
27. FULLER, E. M.: Injury-prone children. *Am. J. Orthopsychiat., 18*:708-723 (Oct.) 1948.
28. GIBERSON, L. G.: Practical value and application of industrial health work from viewpoint of psychiatry. *Indust. Med., 9*:626-629 (Dec.) 1940.
29. GREENWOOD, M., AND WOODS, H. M.: The incidence of industrial accidents with special reference to multiple accidents. (Medical Research Committee, Industrial Fatigue Research Report No. 4) London, His Majesty Stationary Office, 1919.
30. ——— AND YULE, G. U.: An inquiry into the nature of frequency distributions representative of multiple happenings. *J. R. Statist. Soc., Lond., 83*:255, 1920.
31. HERSEY, REXFORD B.: *"Bio-rhythmic" studies.* Philadelphia, Univ. of Penn. Press, 1932.

32. HEYMAN, H.: Significance of accidents and their prevention. *Wien. med. Wchnschr., 93:*453-459 (Aug. 14) 1943.
33. HILDEBRANDT, H. AND ROSS, K.: Individual affinity to accidents. *Veroff. Medverwalt., 36:*211-313, 1932.
34. HORN, D.: A study of pilots with repeated aircraft accidents. *J. Aviation Med., 18:*440-449, 1947.
35. JOHNSON, H. M.: The detection and treatment of accident-prone drivers. *Psychol. Bull., 43:*489-532, 1946.
36. KEMP, W. N.: Human hazards in industrial employment. *Occup. Med., 5:*729-738, (June) 1948.
36A. KIRK, E. J.: Hypertension in industry. *J. Indust. Hyg. & Toxicol., 9:*314, (Nov.) 1931.
37. KLEIN, M.: The psychoanalysis of children, London, Hogarth Press, 1932.
38. KUNKLE, E. G.: The psychological background of "pilot error" in aircraft accidents. *J. Aviation Med., 17:*533-567, 1946.
38A. LARSON, J. C.: STEVENSON, H. L., HAGOPIAN, R., STERN, J. I. AND WILLIAMSON, H. L.: The human element in industrial accident prevention, Center for Safety Education, Division of General Education, New York University, New York, N. Y., 1955.
39. MARBE, K.: Praktische Psychologie der Unfalle und Betriebschaden. *Munchen med. Wchnschr.,* 1926.
40. MAURO, V.: The human elements as the cause of industrial accidents. *Folia Med., 33:*453, 1950.
41. McCANCE, R. A. *et al.*: Physical and emotional periodicity in women. *J. Hyg., 37:*571-605 (Oct.) 1937.
42. MENNINGER, K. A.: Purposive accidents as an expression of self-destructive tendencies. *Internat. J. Psycho-Analysis, 17:*6-16 (Jan.) 1936.
43. ———: *Man Against Himself.* New York, Harcourt, Brace & Co., 1938.
44. MILLER, W. G. AND ROSS, T. F.: Aortic size, status lymphaticus and accidental death. *J. Path. & Bact., 54:*455-460 (Oct.) 1942.
45. MURPHY, J. P. H.: Accidents and injuries. *M. Ann. District of Columbia, 3:*1-7 (Jan.) 1934.
46. NEWBOLD, E. M.: Contribution to the study of the human factor in the causation of accidents. Indust. Health Research Board. Rep. No. 34, 1926.
47. ———: Practical applications to the statistics of repeated events. *J. R. Statist. Soc., Lond., 90:*487-547, 1927.

48. OSBORNE, E. E. AND VERNON, H. M.: The influence of temperature and other conditions on the frequency of industrial accidents. Indust. Fatigue Research Board, Rep. No. 19, 1-17, 1922.
49. PUTNAM, J. J. AND STEVENS, M.: A study of the mental life of the child. *Psychoanalyt. Rev.*, 5:514-515, 1918.
50. RAWSON, A. J.: Accident proneness. *Psychosom. Med.* 6:88-94 (Jan.) 1944.
51. RUPP, F. AND BATTEY, ALVAND: *Hurt at Home.* Works Prog. Admin. Proj. No. 2950, sponsored by the Cook County Bureau of Public Welfare and supervised by the National Safety Council (Aug.) 1936.
52. SCHMIDEBERG, M.: A note of suicide. *Internat. J. Psycho-Analysis*, 17:1-5, 1936.
53. SCHULZINGER, M. S.: Accident Syndrome-A Clinical Approach. *A.M.A. Arch. Indust. Health*, 11:66-71, (Jan.) 1955; *Nat. Safety News*, 70:116 (Oct.) 1954.
54. ———: Accident Syndrome-A Clinical Approach, Intensive Twenty-Year Study of 35,000 Consecutive Accidental Injuries. *A.M.A. Arch. Indust. Hyg. & Surg.*, 10:426-433 (Nov.) 1954.
55. ———: Accident Proneness. *Indust. Med. & Surg.*, 23:151 (April) 1954; *Nat. Safety News*, 69:32 (June) 1954.
56. ———: The Incidence of Accidents in Relation to the Annual Cycle. *Indust. Med. & Surg.*, 22:49 (Feb.) 1953.
57. SLOCOMBE, C. S. AND BINGHAM, W. V.: Individual differences in industrial personnel. *Eugenic News*, 15: 1930; *Personnel J.*, 6:7 and 25, 1926.
58. SODDY, K.: Psychologic aspects of accidents and accident prevention. *Brit. M. J.*, 2:623-626 (Oct. 18) 1947.
59. SUTTER, R. A.: Accidents—the cancer of industry. *Indust. Med. & Surg.*, 19:31-34 (Jan.) 1950.
60. VERNON, H. M.: *Accidents and their Prevention.* New York, Cambridge Univ. Press, 1936.
61. ———: *Health in Relation to Occupation.* New York, Oxford Med. Publ., 1939.
62. VICARY, W. H.: Accidents, analysis at hospital for psychotic patients, *Med. Bull. Vet. Admin.*, 18:292-296 (Jan.) 1942.
63. VITELES, M. S.: Research in selection of motormen. *J. Personnel Res.* 4:100-115, 1925.
64. WOLFF, E.: Accident proneness; a serious industrial problem. *Indust. Med. & Surg.*, 19:419-426 (Sept.) 1950.

65. WONG, W. A. AND HOBBS, G. E.: Personal factors in industrial accidents. *Indust. Med. & Surg., 18*:291-294 (July) 1949.
66. Division of Labor Statistics and Research of the State of California, Hour of Occurrence of Industrial Injuries. California, 1948.
67. *Encyclopaedia Britannica.* Industrial accidents, *12*:276-290, 1946.
68. Indust. Health Research Board, Industrial health in war. Emergency Rep. No. 1, London, 1940.
69. _____: The personal factor in accidents. Rep. No. 3, London, 1942.
70. National Research Council, Committee on Work in Industry, *Fatigue of Workers.* New York, Reinhold Publishing Co., 1941.
71. National Safety Council, *Accident facts.* Chicago, Ill., annual.
72. BROWN, E. W. AND GHISELLI, E. E.: Accident proneness among streetcar motormen and motor coach operators. *J. Appl. Psychol., 32*:20-23 (Feb.) 1948.
73. COBB, P. W.: The limit of usefulness of accident rate as a measure of accident proneness. *J. Appl. Psychol., 24*:154-159, 1940.

INDEX

A

Abdomen, injuries to, 16
  industrial, 113
  non-industrial, 115
Abrasions
  in industry, 110, 111
  non-industrial, 112
Accidents
  age and, 11, 12, 18, 176. *See also*
    Age
  causation of, 182
    concepts of, 34
      history, 34
    dread of injury in, 161
    emotions in, 172
    environment and, 163
    mental maladjustments and, 11, 190
      factors in, 166
    physical defects in, 161
    psychological factors in, 180
  causative factors, types of, 50
  causes of, 15, 17, 109, 166
    self-destruction theory, 41, 42
  classes of, 109
  clinical medical approach to, 206
  correlation between major and minor, 151
  cyclical pattern of, 11, 212
    in children, 11
  death rate in, 16, 109, 180, 210
  definition, Introduction
  distribution of, theoretical, 150
  epidemics of, 17
  epidemiology, 6, 8
  etiology of, 34, 35
  fortuity and, 16
  frequency, 16
    hypertension and, 197
    sickness related to, 4
  "habit," 38, 182
  hourly distribution of, 11, 29, 33, 79-86, 124-134. *See also* Diurnal cycle
  incidence, *See* Age, Hour, Industrial, Maladjustment, Month, Multiple, Non-industrial, Sex, Season
  industrial, *See* Industrial accidents
  injuries in, Introduction
  liability, 40
  maladjustment and, 14, 164, 190. *See also* Group B
  mean frequency, 151
  moods and, 202
  motive in, 41
  neurosis, 59
  non-industrial, *See* Non-industrial accidents
  in physically handicapped, 200
  prevention, Preface, 184, 215, 217, 218
    education and, 184
    medical examinations and, 189
    psychological factors in, 180, 184
  principal classes, Introduction
  probability, 213
  proneness, Introduction, 13, 14, 21, 35, 39, 49, 50, 175, 182, 183, 222
    benefits derived in 47
    in children, 56
    classification of, 54
    development of, 58
    history of, 35
    measurability of, 39
    personality profile of, 44, 55
    in pilots, 52
    prediction of, 50
    psychological aspects of, 42
    relative degrees of, 178
  prospective, 170
  from psychological conflicts, 58
  repetition, 13. *See also* Repetition and Multiple accidents
  responsibility for, Introduction
  seasons and, 11. *See also* Months and Annual Cycle

syndrome, Introduction, Frontispiece, 17, 160
    diagnosis of, 214
    elements of, 215
    time and, 11
        peak hour for, 11
    weather and, 11
    without human injury, Introduction
Ackerman, N. W., 35, 38, 40, 47, 56, 219
Adelstein, A. M., 151, 219
Adjustment and, *See* Group A and Group B
Adler, A., 40, 52, 219
Age
    accidents and, 11, 18, 176, 211
        aggressive, 64, 65
        children's, 56
        falls, 63
        from foreign bodies, 66
        handling objects, 62
        household utensils, 61
        industrial, 75, 76, 84, 85, 88, 89, 110, 111, 113, 116, 120, 122, 123, 136, 140, 141, 146
            female, 78, 128, 130, 131
            male, 77, 127, 129, 131
            patients, 142
        motor vehicles, 67, 100, 101, 102
        non-industrial, 70, 71, 72, 87, 88, 90, 95, 96, 97, 98, 99, 112, 115, 116, 117, 118, 120, 121, 125, 136, 145
            female, 73
        multiple, 91, 92, 148, 149
        population, 153
        stumbling, 68
    distribution
        correlation of, 155
        differences between, 156, 157, 158, 159
        in illness, 20, 94, 152
Aggression, accidents from, 64, 65
Aggressive behavior
    accidents due to, 14, 15
    in accident patients, 173
    non-industrial, 117, 118
Aircraft accidents, "pilot error" in, 52
Aisenson, M. R., 201, 219
Alexander, F., 55, 219
Amputations
    industrial, 110, 111
    non-industrial, 112
Ankles, injuries to, 16
    industrial, 113
    non-industrial, 115
Annual cycle, accident incidence and, 11, 26, 28, 69-78, 120-123. *See also* Age, Female, Industrial, Male, Month, Non-industrial, Season
Aorta, size in accidental death, 202
Arbous, A. G., Introduction, 35, 37, 40, 151, 219
Arms, injuries to, 16
    industrial, 113, 114
    non-industrial, 115
August, accident incidence in, 26, 27
Automobile accidents, 187. *See also* Motor vehicle accidents

B

Back, injuries to, 16
    industrial, 113
    non-industrial, 115
Bakwin, H., 58, 219
Bakwin, R. M., 58, 219
Battey, A., 35, 120, 222
Bender, L., 56, 57, 220
Benedek, T., 204, 219
Billings, E. G., 205, 219
Bills, A. G., 199, 219
Bingham, W. V., 197, 222
Bites, animals and human
    industrial, 110, 111
    non-industrial, 112, 117, 118
Body
    areas involved in accidents, 16
    injuries
        industrial, 113, 114, 116
        non-industrial, 115, 116

INDEX

Bond, D. D., 53, 219
Boys, accidents in, 12, 27, 32, 56
British
    Health Industrial Research Board, 196
    Medical Research Council, 37, 223, 175
Brown, E. W., 178
Burns, 109
    fatal, in home, 119
    in industry, 110, 111
    non-industrial, 112

C

California Division of Labor Statistics and Research, 125, 223
Chambers, E. G., 36, 40, 151, 195, 198, 220
Chambers, N. D., 49, 219
Charts, 61-105
Chest, injuries to, 16
    industrial, 113
    non-industrial, 115
"Chi square test of goodness of fit," 9
Chidester, L., 35, 38, 40, 56, 219
Children
    accidents in
        body area injuries in, 17
        cyclical pattern of, 11
        diurnal cycle in, 32, 33
        hours of non-industrial accidents and, 81
        incidence in, 192
        parental adjustment and, 24
        proneness to, 56
        psychodynamics of, 55
        types of, 15
    illness incidence in, 20
Cincinnati
    accident data from, 3
    population, 156, 158, 159
        accidents
            in relation to, 136
            distribution of, 193
            age distribution, 153

Cobb, P. W., 14, 178, 182
Compensation, industrial injuries and, 114
Contusions
    industrial, 110, 111
    non-industrial, 112
Correlation, rank order, 10
Csillag, I., 16, 54, 219
Culpin, M., 198, 219, 220

D

Deaths
    accidental, 16, 109, 180, 210
    from falls at home, 119
    instinct in, 42
Denial reaction, in accident patients, 172
Depression cycles, 203
Dermatitis
    contact, in industry, 110, 111
    non-industrial, 112
Dislocations
    in industry, 110, 111
    non-industrial, 112
Diurnal cycle, accident incidence and, 11, 29, 79-86, 124-134. *See also* Age, Female, Hour, Industrial, Male, Multiple accidents, Non-industrial
Drowning, 109
Dunbar, F., 14, 16, 23, 35, 38, 39, 40, 42, 43, 45, 46, 47 51, 52, 177, 183, 220

E

Ears, injuries to, 16
    industrial, 113
    non-industrial, 115
Education, accident prevention and, 184, 188, 217, 218
Elbows, injuries to, 16
    industrial, 113
    non-industrial, 115
Electricity, industrial injuries and, 119

Emotions, accidents and, 43, 172
  industrial, 54
Encyclopaedia Britannica, Introduction, 223
Environment
  abnormal, 163
  in accident syndrome, 11
Environmental hazards, accidents and, 181
Explosives, industrial injuries and, 119
Eye, injuries to, 16
  industrial, 113, 114
  non-industrial, 115

F

Fabian, A. A., 56, 57, 220
Face, injuries to, 16
  industrial, 113
  non-industrial, 115
Falls, 63, 109
  in home, 119
  incidence of, 15
  industrial, 119
  non-industrial, 117, 118
Farmer, E., 36, 40, 151, 195, 198, 220
Fatigue, accidents and, 199, 200
February, accident incidence in, 26, 27, 28
Females
  accidents
    aggressive, 64
    cyclical distribution, 27
    diurnal distribution, 124
    falls, 63
    foreign bodies, 66
    handling objects and, 62
    household utensils and, 61
    incidence of, 12, 14, 19, 20, 176
    industrial, 30, 78, 104, 105, 106, 110, 111, 113, 116, 123, 134, 137, 138, 140, 141, 144
      hours of, 84, 85, 126, 128, 130, 131, 132
      multiple, 137, 138, 140, 141
    motor vehicle, 67, 101, 102
    multiple, 22
      age distribution, differences in, 157
    non-industrial, 73, 87, 90, 95, 103, 105, 108, 112, 115, 116, 118, 133, 134, 145
      hours in, 79, 81, 82, 83, 132
      multiple, 96, 97, 98, 139, 148, 149
    proneness, 38
    stumbling, 68
  illness in, 94, 152
  industrial
    injuries in, 146
      by month, 102
    patients, 142
  non-industrial injuries of, by month, 120, 121
Fetterman, J. L., 50, 51, 220
Fingers, injuries to, 16
  industrial, 113, 114
  non-industrial, 115, 118
Firearms, 109
  fatal, in home, 119
Fires, 109
Foot, injuries to, 16
  industrial, 113
  non-industrial, 113
Forearm, injuries to, 16
  industrial, 113
  non-industrial, 115
Foreign body
  in body orifice
    industrial, 110, 111
    non-industrial, 112
  in eye
    industrial, 110, 111
    non-industrial, 112
Forster, N. K., 50, 220
Fortuity, accidents and, 16
Fractures
  in industry, 110, 111
  non-industrial, 112
  personality studies in, 23
  psychological aspects and, 42

INDEX

Freud, S., 41, 42, 48, 220
Fuller, E. M., 56, 220

G

Genitalia, injuries to, 16
    industrial, 113
    non-industrial, 115
Ghiselli, E. E., 178
Giberson, L. G., 54, 220
Girls, accidents and, 12, 27, 32
Greenwood, M., 35, 36, 37, 38, 39, 150, 182, 220
Group A, normally adjusted, 3, 4, 22, 23, 24, 25, 26, 51, 65, 87, 88, 91, 92, 97, 98, 99, 100, 101, 103, 107, 108, 112, 118, 132, 134, 135, 136, 139, 145, 148, 149, 152, 155, 156, 157, 191, 192, 193
Group B, maladjusted, 4, 22, 23, 24, 25, 26, 65, 87, 88, 91, 92, 97, 98, 99, 100, 102, 103, 107, 108, 112, 118, 132, 134, 135, 136, 139, 145, 148, 149, 152, 155, 156, 157, 190, 191, 192, 193

H

Hagopian, R., 199, 221
Hand, injuries to, 16
    industrial, 113, 114
    non-industrial, 115
Hazards, accidents caused by, 35
Head, injuries to, 16
    industrial, 113, 114, 116
    non-industrial, 115, 116
Health, accidents and, 195
Hedri, E., Jr., 16, 54, 219
Heinrich, H. W., 178
Hersey, R. B., 202, 203, 204, 220
Heyman, H., 39, 182, 221
Hildebrandt, H., 39, 182, 221
Hip, injuries to, 16
    industrial, 113
    non-industrial, 115
Hobbs, G. E., 51, 223
Home accidents, Introduction, 109
    fatal, principal causes of, 119
    hospitalized, causes of, 120
    incidence, 186
Horn, D., 53, 177, 221
Hour. *See also* Diurnal cycle
    correlation between industrial and non-industrial accidents by, 154
    grouping of, non-industrial accidents in, 132
    industrial accidents by, 84, 85, 126, 127, 128, 129, 130, 131, 132
    non-industrial accidents by, 79, 80, 81, 82, 83, 86, 125, 133
Household utensils, accidents and, 61, 188
Human behavior, accidents and, Introduction, 35, 182, 198, 216
Hypertension, accident frequency and, 197

I

Illness
    age
        and sex distribution, 94, 152
        distribution, difference in, 156
    compared to accidents, 20
    correlation between accident frequency and, 195
Indemnity neurosis, 50
Industrial
    accidents, 140, 141, 143
        age in, 18, 74, 75, 76
        distribution
            correlation between, 155
            differences in, 156, 157, 158
        cumulative percentage of, 140
        distribution, 104, 105, 106
        diurnal cycle and, 29, 33, 124, 212
        factors in, 54, 199
        females and, 78. *See also* Female industrial accidents
        frequency, distribution of, 150
        hours of, 84, 85, 126, 127, 128, 129, 130, 131, 132
        2-hour periods of, 134

human hazards in, 53, 200
incidence, 186
males and, 77. *See also* Male industrial accidents
months and, 69, 74, 76, 120. *See also* Annual cycle
multiple, 107, 122, 123, 137, 138, 140, 141, 143
neuropsychiatric aspects of, 51
number per firm, 136
peak hour for, 12
personality studies in, 51
principal causes, 119
ratio of accidents to patients, 144
relation to population, 88, 136
residence and, 135
seasonal incidence, 28, 29, 75, 122
sex distribution in, 19
single, 137, 138, 140, 141
types of
    industry in, 135
    injury in, 110, 111
Health Research Board, 35, 223
injuries, 3
    in consecutive years, 146 147
    hours of, correlation between non-industrial and, 154
    multiple, frequency of recurrence, 147
neurosis, 50, 51
patients, 146
    age, sex, and number of accidents, 142
    ratio to accidents, 144

Industry, types of accidents in, 135

Injuries
    in accidents, 109
    industrial, *See* Industrial injuries
    non-industrial, *See* Non-industrial injuries
    permanent, 16
    self inflicted, in children, 55

Injury neurosis, 50, 51

Intelligence, injuries and, 56

Internal injuries, 16
    industrial, 113
    non-industrial, 115
Irresponsibilty, 164, 216. *See also* Maladjustment
    accident incidence in, 190

J

Jaw, injuries to, 16
    industrial, 113
    non-industrial, 115
Johnson, H. M., 39, 177, 182, 221

K

Kemp, W. N., 53, 221
Kerrich, J. D., 35, 151, 219
Kirk, E. J., 197, 221
Klein, M., 55, 221
Knees, injuries to, 16
    industrial, 113
    non-industrial, 115
Kunkle, E. G., 52, 221

L

Lacerations
    in industry, 110, 111
    non-industrial, 112
Larson, J. C., 199, 221
Legs, injuries to, 16
    industrial, 113, 114
    non-industrial, 115
Lower extremities, injuries to, 16
    industrial, 113, 116
    non-industrial, 115, 116

M

Machinery
    industrial injuries by, 119
    non-industrial injuries by, 118
Maladjustment, 164, 207, 216. *See also* Group B
    accident incidence in, 23, 190
    age in, 24, 25
    in accident victims, 11, 14, 176

medical examination in, 189
psychological elements in, 166
repeated accidents in, 23, 25
Males
   accidents in
      aggressive, 64
      diurnal distribution of, 124
      falls in, 63
      foreign body, 66
      handling objects, 62
      household utensils, 61
      incidence of, 12, 14, 19, 20, 176, 211
      industrial, 30, 77, 104, 105, 106, 110, 111, 113, 116, 134, 137, 138, 140, 141, 143, 144, 146
         hours of, 84, 85, 126, 127, 128, 129, 131, 132
         multiple, 122, 137, 138, 140, 141, 143
      motor vehicle, 67, 101, 102
      multiple, 22
         age distribution differences in, 157
      non-industrial, 72, 87, 90, 112, 115, 116, 118, 133, 134, 145
         correlation between age distribution, 155
         hours in, 79, 81, 82, 83, 132
         months and, 120, 121
         multiple, 96, 97, 98, 139, 148, 149
      stumbling, 68
   accidental death in, 180
   aggressive behavior in, 15
   illness in, 94, 152
   industrial
      injuries, by month, 120
      patients, 142
   medical examinations in, 189
   non-industrial injuries in, 95, 103, 107, 108
Marbe, K., 38, 182, 221
Mauro, V., 198, 211

McCance, R. A., 204, 221
Medical
   approach to accidents, 206
   examinations, in accident prevention, 189
Menninger, K. A., 35, 38, 41, 42, 47, 50, 183, 221
Miller, W. G., 202, 221
Months. *See also* Annual cycle and Season
   accident incidence by, 26, 69
   industrial
      female accidents, 78
      injuries by, 76, 120, 122, 123
      male accidents, 77
   non-industrial injuries by, 120, 121
      female, 73
Mood swings, 202
Motor vehicles
   accidents and, 67, 109
      non-industrial, 100, 101, 102, 117, 118
   injuries in, Introduction, 119
Mouth, injuries to, 16
   industrial, 113
   non-industrial, 115
Multiple accidents, 103, 104, 105, 152, 182, 191, 192. *See also* Repetition
   age distribution
      correlation between, 155
      differences in, 156, 157
   in children, 192, 193
   industrial, 137, 138, 140, 141, 142, 143, 144
      frequency of recurrence, 147
      hours of,
         in female, 131, 132
         in male, 131, 132
   medical examinations in, 189
   non-industrial, 91, 96, 97, 98, 99, 139, 148, 149
      hours of, 132
Murphy, J. P. H., 198, 221

N

National
   Research Council, 39, 182, 223

Safety
  Congress, 37, 175
  Council, Introduction, 35, 109, 114, 119, 223
Neck, injuries to, 16
  industrial, 113, 116
  non-industrial, 113, 116
Neurosis
  accident frequency and, 199
  compensation, 53, 186
  indemnity, 50
  industrial, 50, 51, 53
  inherent, 50
  injury, 50, 51
  traumatic, 186
Newbold, E. M., 35, 40, 195, 196, 197, 221
Non-industrial
  accidents, 145, 149
    age in, 18, 70, 71, 80, 81, 82, 83
      distribution
        correlation between, 155
        differences in, 156
    common types of, 117
    diurnal distribution, 11, 31, 33, 124
    falls in, 63
    foreign bodies, 66
    handling objects and, 62
    hours of, 79, 80, 81, 82, 83, 86, 125, 132, 133
      by 2-hour periods, 134
      correlation between industrial and, 154
    household utensils and, 61
    maladjustment and, 23
    in males, 72
    months and, 69, 70, 72, 120, 121
    multiple, 91, 92, 96, 97, 98, 99, 103, 107, 108, 139, 148, 149
    population
      age distribution of, 153
      relation to, 87, 88, 136
    residence and, 135
    seasonal incidence, 28, 71, 133
    sex distribution, 19
    types of, 15, 118
      injury in, 112
  injuries, 3, 90
Normal adjustment, accidents in, *See* Group A
Nose, injuries to, 16
  industrial, 113
  non-industrial, 115

O

Objects
  stumbling into, non-industrial, 117, 118
  dropping, non-industrial, 117, 118
  falling, industrial, 119
  handling
    industrial, 119
    non-industrial, 117, 118
  stepped on, non-industrial, 118
  striking against, industrial, 119
Osborne, E. E., 29, 31, 222

P

Parental adjustment, in accident-habit children, 56
Peak
  age, for accidents, 176
  hours, for accidents, 32, 33
    in children, 11
    fatigue and, 200
    in females, 13
    for industrial accidents, 12
  year, 12
Perineum, injuries to, 16
  industrial, 113
  non-industrial, 115
Personality, in accidents, 35, 182, 200
  accident-prone, 55
Phalangeal joints, injuries to, 16
  industrial, 113
  non-industrial, 115
"Phallic-narcisistic character," 59

Physical
  environment, accident syndrome and, 163, 216
  handicaps, 200
  impairment, influence on accidents, 161
Physicians, accident prevention and, 185, 189, 218
Poisons, 109
  fatal, in home, 119
  gas, 109, 119
  in industry, 110, 111
  non-industrial, 112
Psychodynamics, 41
  in children, 55
Psychological factors in accidents, 180
Psychological testing, 198, 199, 200
Public (non-motor vehicle) accidents, Introduction, 109
Puncture wounds
  industrial, 110, 111
  non-industrial, 112
Putnam, J. J., 55, 223

R

Railroads, 109
Rank order correlation, 10
Rawson, A. J., 35, 38, 39, 40, 47, 49, 50, 182
Reiser, M. F., 49, 219
Repetition of accidents, 13, 21. *See also* Multiple accidents
  in children, 24
  contributory factors to, 14
  hourly distribution of, 33
  maladjustment and, 23
  personality in, 52, 54
Residence, in accidents, 135
Ross, K., 39, 221
Ross, T. F., 202, 221
Rubenstein, B. B., 204, 219
Rupp, F., 35, 120, 222

S

Sado-masochistic behavior, 57
Safety measures, Preface, 34, 181, 206
  accidents and, 15
Scalp, injuries to, 16
  industrial, 113
  non-industrial, 115
Schmideberg, M., 55, 222
School-hour accidents, 12, 28
Schulzinger, M. S., 210, 222
Season, accident incidence by, 11, 26, 28, 29
  industrial, 75, 122
  non-industrial, 71, 133
Self-destructive tendencies, 41, 47, 48
Sex, *See also* Male and Female
  accident distribution and, 12, 19, 44, 46, 176
  in illness, 20
Shoulders, injuries to, 16
  industrial, 113
  non-industrial, 115
Sickness, accident frequency and, 4
Skeleton, injuries to, 16
  industrial, 113
  non-industrial, 115
Slocombe, C. S., 197, 222
Smith, M., 198, 219
Sociological Studies, 199, 200
Soddy, K., 197, 222
Sprains
  industrial, 110, 111
  non-industrial, 112
Stern, J. I., 199, 221
Stevens, M., 55, 222
Stevenson, H. L., 199, 221
Strains
  industrial, 110, 111
  non-industrial, 112
Stumbling, accidents from, 68
Suffocation, mechanical, fatal in home, 119
Suicidal tendencies, 55
Summer, accidents in, 11, 12, 26, 27, 28
Susceptibility, 13, 218
  health and, 195
  sex distribution in, 19
Sutter, R. A., 54, 222
Syndrome, accident, 160. *See also* Accident syndrome

T

"T" test, 10
Tables, 106-159
Teeth, injuries to, 16
   industrial, 113
   non-industrial, 115
Tendons, severed
   industrial, 110, 111
   non-industrial, 112
Thigh, injuries to, 16
   industrial, 113
   non-industrial, 115
Time, accidents and, 11
Toes, injuries to, 16
   industrial, 113, 114
   non-industrial, 115
Tools
   industrial injuries by, 119
   non-industrial injuries by, 118
Traumatophilic diathesis theory, 42, 48, 59
Trigger episode, 168, 216
   behavior in presence of, 169
Trunk, injuries to, 16
   industrial, 113, 116
   non-industrial, 115, 116

U

Universal risk, 161, 216
Upper extremity, injuries to, 16
   industrial, 113, 116
   non-industrial, 115, 116

V

Vernon, H. M., 29, 31, 35, 40, 150, 177, 178, 197, 199, 222
Vicary, W. H., 197, 222
Viteles, M. S., 201, 222

W

Weather, accidents and, 11
Williamson, H. L., 221
Winter, accidents in, 11, 12, 26
Wolff, E., 93, 123, 222
Wong, W. A., 51, 223
Woods, H. M., 35, 36, 37, 38, 39, 150, 182, 220
Work material, exploration of, 3
Wrists, injuries to, 16
   industrial, 113
   non-industrial, 115

Y

Yule, G. U., 35, 150, 220

This Book

THE ACCIDENT SYNDROME

By

Morris S. Schulzinger, M.A., M.D.

was set and printed by The Marvin D. Evans Company of Fort Worth, Texas. It was bound by The Becktold Company of St. Louis, Missouri. The engravings were made by G. R. Grubb and Company of Champaign, Illinois. The page trim size is 6 x 9 inches. The type page is 26 x 43 picas. The type face is Linotype Janson, set 11 point on 13 point. The text paper is 70-lb. Garamond Eggshell. The cover is Bancroft's Linen Finish 6445.

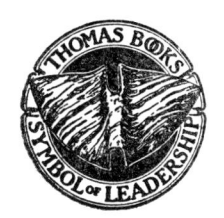

With THOMAS BOOKS *careful attention is given to all details of manufacturing and design. It is the Publisher's desire to present books that are satisfactory as to their physical qualities and artistic possibilities and appropriate for their particular use.* THOMAS BOOKS *will be true to those laws of* quality *that assure a good name and good will.*